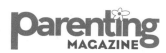

D1370781

Pregnancy
planner

Ziba Kashef and the editors of *Parenting* magazine

CHRONICLE BOOKS

SAN FRANCISCO

About *Parenting* The premier U.S. magazine for moms, *Parenting* magazine provides honest, real-world advice on raising children and the emotional support and connection moms need to enjoy their full lives. Founded in 1987, *Parenting* remains the cornerstone of The Parenting Group family, which includes Parenting.com and *Conceive* and *Babytalk* magazines.

About the Author A San Francisco–based writer who specializes in women's and children's health issues, Ziba Kashef wrote this book while pregnant with her second child. Formerly, she was editor in chief at *Pregnancy* magazine, editor at *Bay Area Parent*, and a senior editor at *Parenting* and *Sesame Street Parents*. She has written for BabyCenter.com, and authored the book *Backyards for Kids*.

Acknowledgments Special thanks to *Parenting* magazine staff: Susan Kane, editor in chief; Elizabeth Anne Shaw, executive editor; Stephanie Wood, deputy editor; and Lisa Moran, former *Babytalk* editor in chief. Thanks to Weldon Owen staff: Roger Shaw, VP/publisher; Elizabeth Dougherty, executive editor; Sarah Gurman, assistant editor; Katharine Moore, editorial assistant; Kelly Booth, associate creative director; Renée Myers, senior designer; Meghan Hildebrand and Michel Gadwa, designers; Chris Hemesath, production director; and Michelle Duggan, production manager. Also thanks to Julie Feinstein Adams, project editor; Denise Schipani, contributing editor; Ann Sackrider, researcher; Gaye Allen, design consultant; and Miranda Gregory, editorial intern.

Weldon Owen Inc.
415 Jackson Street
San Francisco, CA 94111
www.weldonowen.com

ISBN 978-0-8118-7132-7

Manufactured in China

10 9 8 7 6 5 4 3 2 1

Chronicle Books LLC
680 Second Street
San Francisco, CA 94107
www.chroniclebooks.com

what's inside...

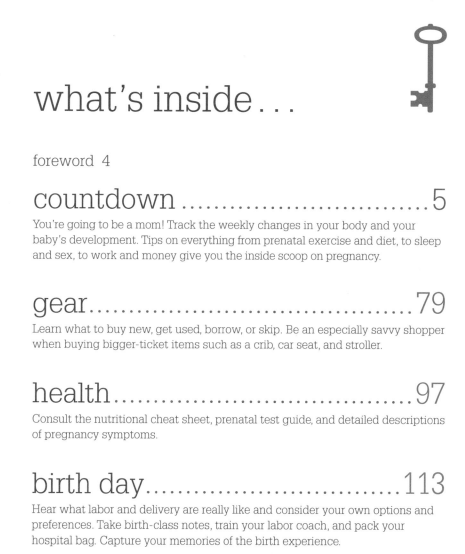

foreword

Let the countdown begin! In nine months—or sooner—you'll be a mom. You may not feel all that different just yet, but you will! Every single day, your body is undergoing dramatic (and sometimes downright weird) changes—all while your baby-to-be is developing in remarkable ways.

As editors at *Parenting* magazine and moms, we're thrilled to offer this *Pregnancy Planner,* your one-stop organizer, journal, and month-by-month information source.

In the first section, Countdown, we'll track your pregnancy with you, dishing out practical tips, timely reminders, and insight into what you and your baby are going through right now. We've also left space on the pages for you to jot down observations, feelings, questions for your doctor, to-do lists, whatever you like. Gear will help you navigate the dizzying array of baby accoutrements. The final sections focus on your well-being (Health), labor and delivery (Birth Day), and what to expect after the big event (Homecoming).

This is not meant to be a coffee table tome! Slip it into your purse and take it with you to prenatal visits, pediatrician interviews, shopping trips—as well as to the hospital on the big day. Later on, when the blur (and sleep deprivation!) of new motherhood makes your pregnancy memories fuzzy, you can pull out your *Pregnancy Planner* and reread your own notes about this amazing nine-month journey.

Susan Kane
Parenting Editor-in-Chief

countdown

countdown

You're pregnant! Congratulations! Whether your good news is a surprise or very well planned, whether it took months or one lucky night, you're about to embark on an extraordinary journey. It's normal to feel both thrilled and nervous in equal measures. Your body and your life are going to change in ways you expect and in ways you probably can't imagine.

The Countdown section offers a place to track and record this journey as a mom-to-be. (Pregnancy dating begins on the first day of your last menstrual period, so this section starts with week 5—around the earliest point when you can see that plus sign on a pregnancy test.) Write a little or a lot, paste in belly photos and baby ultrasounds, or just read the news of the week and take a nap.

How did you find out you were pregnant?

_____

_____

How did you feel when you learned the result?

_____

_____

How did you tell your partner?

_____

_____

How do you feel about being pregnant?

_____

_____

brain-booster

In addition to taking prenatal vitamins, ask your doctor about taking a docosahexaenoic acid (DHA) supplement. This fatty acid helps a baby's brain and nerve cells develop. DHA is found in fatty fish such as salmon (see page 98 for info about eating fish). There are also nutrition bars with DHA made especially for pregnant women.

don't panic!

Downed a drink or two before you learned you were expecting? Don't worry. A little bit of alcohol in those early days is not likely to present a problem. What's most important now is to pass on all alcohol from here on out.

pop those vitamins

If you aren't already taking a prenatal vitamin, start now. (Your doctor can prescribe one or recommend an over-the-counter brand.) It's important to get 400 to 600 µg (micrograms) of folic acid daily to help prevent neural tube defects. A prenatal vitamin should also have 27 mg of iron (talk to your doctor before taking any additional iron supplements).

One glitch: Prenatal vitamins make some moms-to-be queasy or make morning sickness worse. If that happens, ask your doctor about vitamins that may be easier to digest, try different brands, and experiment with taking your vitamin with food or at night. Look for one where the daily dose is several pills that you can take at different times during the day.

Ask your doctor about taking an extra calcium supplement. If you take one, be sure to take it at a different time during the day than your prenatal vitamin, since calcium can inhibit iron absorption.

off the menu

Sorting out what you should and shouldn't eat during pregnancy can be overwhelming. Here are some tips; see pages 98 to 99 for a detailed cheat sheet and page 8 for information about caffeine.

❖ Fish is one of the most confusing categories, making consulting a species-specific list (page 98) nearly essential. In general, avoid fish with high mercury levels, farm-raised fish, raw fish, and smoked refrigerated seafood.

❖ What's safe? Up to 12 ounces (340 g) of fish with low mercury levels, such as canned or wild salmon, per week. Salmon is packed with essential fatty acids too. Limit your intake of canned light tuna to 6 ounces (170 g) per week of the allowed 12 ounces but avoid albacore ("white") tuna.

❖ Skip any raw and unpasteurized dairy products and soft cheeses, such as Brie or feta. Also avoid unpasteurized juices (think: fresh-pressed apple juice), raw sprouts, and uncooked food made with raw eggs, such as some salad dressings.

❖ Heat deli meats and hotdogs until steaming hot before eating.

week 5

you

- You're most likely still fitting in your favorite jeans, but your breasts are already feeling tender and full.

- Growing a baby is exhausting work for your body. Heed any cues to cut yourself some slack and rest, rest, rest.

your baby

- The embryo is smaller than an apple seed. The cluster of cells that will become your baby's heart has formed and is beating. The brain and spinal cord are taking shape.

- The placenta and umbilical cord are already forming, and will soon be passing oxygen and nutrients from you to your baby.

"I first realized I might be pregnant when my husband and I rented a movie and I had to pause it about six or seven times so I could use the bathroom. I figured I was either pregnant or something was seriously wrong with me!"

no more coffee breaks?

Caffeine inhibits your body's absorption of iron, an important nutrient for fetal development, and some research suggests that a daily 12-ounce (.35 l) or larger cup of coffee may boost the risk of miscarriage. While you don't have to totally give up caffeine, you'll want to keep your intake to fewer than 200 mg a day.

❖ An 8-ounce (.24 l) cup of coffee has about 150 mg of caffeine. If you regularly drink coffee, cut down—or switch to decaf.

❖ Consider drinking a latte. A 12-ounce latte at a popular chain has 75 mg of caffeine—and you get calcium from the milk.

❖ A 12-ounce can of soda has about 50 mg of caffeine. Check the label of energy drinks for caffeine content, too.

❖ An 8-ounce cup of black tea has about 40 mg of caffeine. Green tea also has caffeine, but you'll want to avoid it during your first trimester and drink only moderate amounts later for a different reason: Too much green tea can lower the efficacy of folic acid.

❖ Chocolate is caffeinated, but you'd have to eat a lot of it to get amped. Dark chocolate has about 20 mg per ounce (28 g); milk chocolate has up to 6 mg.

minimizing medicine

If you take prescription medication, tell the prescribing doctor that you're pregnant right away—before making any changes to your drug regime. Also inform your ob-gyn that you're on medication. Some drugs, such as most acne-fighting medicines, aren't recommended during pregnancy, but others are fine to continue taking—and some are essential for your health.

Ask your ob-gyn before taking any over-the-counter medication—even ones for a minor health problem, such as a cold. For example, acetaminophen is fine for aches and pains, but don't take aspirin or ibuprofen—both can affect fetal circulation.

If you come down with a cold or suffer from allergies, using a saline spray or a hot-mist vaporizer might provide some sinus relief. Be wary of herbal remedies during pregnancy; not enough is known about their safety.

not so sweet

Even though artificial sweeteners, like sucralose and aspartame, have not been shown to cause harm to babies in utero, they have no nutritional value. Consider replacing diet drinks with healthier options such as water, skim milk, and juice.

spot check

Notice some spotting? About 20 to 30 percent of women experience mild bleeding in their first trimester, which can vary in color from red to brown. It's usually not cause for concern, but check with your doctor to be sure.

week 6

you

❖ Like more than half of moms-to-be, you may be suffering from some degree of nausea. (See page 10 for what to do.)

❖ Don't be surprised by an increased need to pee: Your growing uterus is already pressing on your bladder. You may even leak a little urine when you laugh or cough. (See page 52 for exercises that could help.)

your baby

❖ Your baby's heart, no bigger than a poppy seed, is beating.

❖ Small cups that are beginning to appear on either side of your baby's forebrain will become eyes.

"I was plagued with stuffy noses and sinus headaches during my two pregnancies. I couldn't take the usual meds since I was preggers, and the rest I couldn't take because I'm allergic to them. So colds were treated only with lemon and honey teas and saltwater gargles, and headaches with compresses and Tylenol."

pack in protein

Your baby needs protein to grow! A pregnant woman requires 60 grams a day. A 3-ounce (85-g) serving—about the size of a deck of cards—of lean poultry, beef, pork, or fish (see page 98 for a list of fish to avoid) has about 15 to 20 grams of protein. You can also get protein from low-fat dairy, eggs, peanut butter, tofu, legumes, and beans.

stay out of the litter box

Cat-litter duty is off limits during pregnancy. Feline fecal matter may harbor *toxoplasma gondii*, a parasite that can cross the placenta and harm your baby. It's rare, but why take the chance if someone else can keep kitty's box clean for now? Gardening is out for the same reason.

going up the scale

You have to do it: Gaining weight during pregnancy is part of the program. The extra weight ensures your baby's growth and your body's ability to carry a fetus. Your ob-gyn will help you determine what's a healthy range of pounds for you to gain and will monitor your weight at each prenatal visit.

The American College of Obstetricians and Gynecologists recommends the following weight gain during pregnancy:

❖ 25 to 35 pounds (11 to 16 kg) for normal-weight women

❖ 28 to 40 pounds (13 to 18 kg) for women who are underweight

❖ 15 to 25 pounds (7 to 11 kg) for those who are overweight

On average, that means you should aim to gain about 3 to 5 pounds (1 to 2 kg) in the first trimester, and about 1 pound (.5 kg) a week in both the second and third trimesters.

There's a fine balance between gaining enough and not too much weight. The downside of putting on too many pounds is increased risk for complications, such as preterm birth and cesarean delivery. Packing on the pounds very quickly early on may be a sign of other maternal health issues, such as gestational diabetes; check in with your doctor if your numbers are spiraling upward.

feeling queasy?

Unfortunately, "morning" sickness can strike at any time of day. Most pregnant women also say they are turned off by certain foods. Here are a few tips that might help.

❖ Eat mini-meals that include protein throughout the day. An empty stomach and low blood sugar can exacerbate nausea.

❖ Carry food with you at all times: crackers, bananas, raw almonds—eating snacks frequently can keep nausea at bay.

❖ Drink ginger tea or ginger ale, grate fresh ginger into a beverage, or chew ginger candy to help soothe an upset stomach.

❖ Check with your doctor to find out if a vitamin B6 supplement might help ease your symptoms.

week 7

you

❖ At your first prenatal visit, you will have a pelvic exam, Pap smear, urine test, and possibly an ultrasound (see page 104 for more about prenatal visits).

❖ Routine blood tests include anemia, Rh factor, and rubella immunity, unless you've been tested recently (see page 106).

your baby

❖ Your baby is about ½ inch (just over 1 cm) from crown to rump, about the size of a raspberry.

❖ Dark spots on her head mark where her eyes and nostrils will be.

❖ Arm buds and legs are starting to form, making her look more like a real baby.

mom to mom

"Just the thought of food made me nauseous. And I love food. Because I never wanted to eat, all of my food choices were out of necessity to give my baby nutrients. I still gained 30 pounds [13.6 kg], but if I hadn't had 24-hour morning sickness, there's no telling how big I would have been!"

the skinny on skin care

Pregnancy hormones can wreak havoc on your skin, causing more oil and breakouts, or less oil and itching—not to mention increased sensitivity to the sun either way. Now that everything you do, you do for two, your skin-care regimen might need a revamp. (Also see page 46.)

❖ Are pimples popping up? It's okay to use products that contain glycolic acid but avoid ingredients that could affect your baby, such as alpha-hydroxy acids, salicylic acid, retinols, or steroids.

❖ If your skin's oil production goes down instead of up, you may be feeling dry and itchy. Drinking more water, taking warm rather than hot showers or baths, using a moisturizing cleanser, and applying body oil right after bathing can help.

❖ Some pregnant women develop dark patches of skin, called the "mask of pregnancy" (officially known as *chloasma* or *melasma*), after sun exposure. To help avoid it, apply broad-spectrum sunscreen (SPF 30 or higher) every day.

savvy smiles

Your blood volume increases during pregnancy, bringing more blood to the gums and causing swelling, sensitivity to bacteria, and possible infection. While your gums most likely will bleed some, watch out for excessive bleeding. This may be a sign of gum disease, which can increase your risk of premature birth. (If you're concerned, check with your dentist.)

To protect your mouth and your baby, brush your teeth and tongue with a soft toothbrush twice a day. Better yet, grab that toothbrush after every meal. Also floss and try to rinse with mouthwash once a day. Stick to your regular schedule if you're due for a cleaning, but skip X-rays.

As for cosmetic procedures like tooth-whitening: Save them for later. Even over-the-counter products haven't been deemed perfectly safe for pregnancy.

painted nails

Dying for a mani-pedi? It's safe, as long as you take some extra precautions. Bring your own tools (nail file, cuticle clipper, etc.) to a salon to reduce infection risk. Opt for a salon with an air-conditioning or air-filtering system that clears out chemical odors. If you do your own nails, apply polish in a well-ventilated area.

show your roots

While all the available research suggests that coloring your hair during pregnancy is safe, it's a good idea to be extra cautious and wait until you're out of the first trimester, when most of the major organ development happens.

week 8

you

❖ Your uterus has grown from the size of a lemon to the size of a tennis ball.

❖ As your uterus enlarges, you may feel occasional cramping in your lower abdomen and sides.

your baby

❖ Your baby is about ¾ inch (2 cm) from crown to rump.

❖ His heart has divided into right and left chambers and beats at 160 to 170 times per minute—twice the rate of an adult's heart.

❖ His eyelids, nose tip, and upper lip are discernible.

mom to mom

"This baby will be my third—my boys are 12 and 16 now. At dinner with my sons and my husband the day I found out I was pregnant, I just went ahead and announced, 'I'm having a baby.' My husband was so surprised he said, 'A baby what?'"

let's get physical

Regular physical activity can rev flagging energy levels and help prime your body for the demands of pregnancy and labor. (For more about exercising while you're pregnant, see page 36.)

❖ If you're already exercising, definitely don't quit! You can often safely maintain your current fitness routine with commonsense modifications as your body changes.

❖ Not much of an exercise fan before now? Get the green light from your obstetrician before starting up. A simple walking routine is a good place to begin.

❖ For pregnancy-specific toning and stretching, take a prenatal yoga, aquatic, or exercise class.

❖ Pregnant women tend to overheat more easily. Take frequent water breaks and ease up before you reach the point where you get short of breath.

❖ Avoid contact sports, such as soccer. Because balance is an increasingly difficult task as you get bigger, skip activities, such as skating or bike riding, that require balance and put you at risk for falls. Stationary bikes are okay.

feeling more than blue?

Many pregnant women report some form of moodiness, irritability, and anxious thoughts. If you have the "pregnancy blues," yoga, meditation, breathing techniques, or support from other pregnant women or veteran moms can help.

However, about 1 in 10 pregnant women will suffer from actual depression, which has physical as well as emotional effects. Symptoms may include persistent sad, empty, or anxious feelings; irritability; overeating or appetite loss; insomnia or excessive sleeping; loss of interest in activities once considered pleasurable; restlessness; inability to make decisions; and feelings of guilt, hopelessness, or worthlessness.

If you think you might be depressed, don't hesitate to consult your doctor. Proper treatment, such as talk therapy and/or medication, is important to your health—and your baby's.

week 9

you

❖ Some lucky women may notice queasiness and fatigue easing up a bit around now.

❖ Bra tight? Cup size can increase more than once during pregnancy. Try a bra extender (see page 26) or go lingerie shopping.

your baby

❖ You can now officially call your embryo a *fetus,* which comes from Latin, meaning "offspring."

❖ About 1 inch (2.5 cm) from crown to rump, she's about the size of a strawberry.

❖ Your baby's joints are mostly formed and are now bending and flexing.

mom to mom

"I walked a lot and stretched to stay flexible, but I let my body relax and, for the first time in years, didn't kill myself at the gym all the time. It was wonderful to let go and eat right and stay active without feeling obsessed or neurotic about it. I was careful not to eat junk food and gain too much weight, but I ate all the healthy food I wanted, moved when I felt like it, and allowed myself to relax and rest more than I ever had."

wash your hands

Doctors advise pregnant women to be extra vigilant about their health. An easy preventative measure: wash your hands often with soap and water. Also try to steer clear of people who aren't feeling well.

vaccine season

If you will be pregnant during flu season, which runs from October through March, be sure to get a flu shot. It will decrease your chance of illness and the pregnancy complications that can arise. Flu vaccines contain traces of egg—if you have an allergy, check with your doctor first. Also, confirm that the shot is mercury-free.

prenatal tests 101

Optional prenatal tests for chromosomal and genetic disorders will be offered in the coming weeks. (For a detailed list of tests, see pages 106 to 109.)

❖ Some tests are screening tests. A positive result indicates an increased risk for disorders, not a diagnosis. Also, false positives are common, especially if you're older. The first-trimester screen, for example, measures the risk of certain chromosomal defects, including Down syndrome. Performed between weeks 11 to 14, this screening test combines a blood test with an ultrasound that measures the amount of fluid at the back of the baby's neck (called "nuchal translucency").

❖ Other tests are diagnostic tests. A positive result indicates if a chromosomal or genetic disorder is actually present. Chorionic villus sampling (CVS), which is performed between weeks 10 and 12, involves removing a small piece of placental tissue from the uterus to test for disorders such as cystic fibrosis. Typically performed between weeks 15 and 20, amniocentesis involves removing a small amount of fluid from the sac around the baby to examine for evidence of problems such as spina bifida.

what you can control

Having prenatal tests is stressful. Not only do you worry about the outcome, but sometimes you're taking a risk just having the procedure. CVS and amniocentesis involve a risk of miscarriage (1 in 100 for CVS and 1 in 200–400 for amnio). After tests, you often have to wait days or weeks for the results.

You do have some control. Prenatal tests are optional. Depending on your age and medical history, your health-care provider may recommend certain ones. Consider the risks—including your emotional state—and potential results carefully. Discuss options with your partner, your physician, and, if available, a genetic counselor to decide what's right for you.

The vast majority of test results come back indicating a healthy baby. If screening results indicate a problem, however, you can consider having a diagnostic test to confirm it or not.

week 10

you

❖ Pregnancy hormones can put your emotions on a hair trigger, so don't be surprised to find yourself sobbing over TV commercials one minute, and snapping at your partner the next. (See page 14.)

❖ You can blame hormones for sleep disturbances, too—which can make you feel even more volatile.

your baby

❖ About 1½ inches (4 cm) from crown to rump, he's about the size and shape of a cocktail shrimp.

❖ Your baby's brain is beginning to grow rapidly, producing nearly 250,000 neurons every minute.

❖ He now has fingers and toes on each hand and foot.

"I'm dying to get that first ultrasound done! Other than typical signs and symptoms—gas, nausea, sore breasts, et cetera—it still doesn't feel real. I just want to see the tiny little blob in there."

pump iron

Your body needs almost twice as much iron when you're pregnant. Iron-rich foods include lean red meat, whole-grain breads, and iron-fortified cereals. Combining veggies with vitamin C–rich food, like spinach and lemon juice, makes it easier for your body to absorb the iron. Your prenatal vitamin also provides iron (see page 6).

weighing in

When it comes to your weight, it's smart to gain slowly and steadily. Don't panic if the scale barely budges during the first trimester, when nausea may make eating more difficult. You'll make up for it later. Also, you might have growth spurts when you gain several pounds in a short period and then level off. Just make sure that you and your doctor are keeping an eye on your overall weight gain.

feeling hot?

This could be your lucky week: Nausea's on the wane, energy is on the rise, and surging estrogen is heating up your libido, with increased circulation sending more blood to your breasts, labia, and clitoris. This engorgement may have you tingling, and the pregnancy hormone oxytocin is stoking the flames of your lust. Your partner's digging your bigger boobs (and so are you!). Your orgasms are bigger and better than ever. You can't get enough. Pregnancy sex can be awesome! (Or not—see below.)

just (don't) do it

Nausea, exhaustion, aching breasts, and a constant urge to pee: It's not surprising that many moms-to-be find their libidos go limp, especially during the first trimester. Even more bad news: The same engorgement that titillates some women can result in a dulling sensation for others.

❖ Maybe you're physically ready for sex, but fears about harming the baby are putting the brakes on your drive? Good news: Your baby is well protected inside the uterus and by the amniotic sac that surrounds him.

❖ But what if one of you simply isn't in the mood for the full mambo? If you're up to it, consider trying some alternate moves: Intimate talk and a creative massage may do the trick.

❖ Prefer to skip body contact altogether? Go ahead. Pregnancy sex tends to get better during the second trimester when nausea generally abates, breasts are often less tender, and physical stamina improves (see description above for inspiration).

week 11

you

❖ Your uterus has expanded to fill your pelvis.

❖ Although your baby may already be kicking, you probably won't feel it for several more weeks.

❖ Between now and week 13, you may have a first-trimester combined screening test performed (see page 108).

your baby

❖ Your baby is about the length of your thumb.

❖ Her head is so big it takes up almost half of her body, and a clear outline of her spine is visible.

❖ She now has the ability to swallow, and her fingernails have started to grow.

"There would be days I couldn't wait till my husband got home so we could get down and dirty, but, as I got closer to the end of the pregnancies, my sex drive would be halted for some reason. But when we did have sex, it was amazing! I would get this tingling sensation all over my body. Your body senses things in a totally different way when you are pregnant."

boy, girl, or surprise?

Your baby's gender will most likely be visible in an ultrasound during the second trimester—and you can get the news even earlier from other tests. So now's the time to decide, if you haven't already, if you want to know the sex of your baby or if you'd rather it be a surprise.

For some parents, the decision is a no-brainer: They're too excited to wait. On the practical side, knowing "boy" or "girl" makes things like picking a name and picking out baby clothes much easier. Still, there are many moms and dads who would rather learn the old-fashioned way—at the birth. Whichever you choose, be prepared: Everyone else will want to know whether you're finding out, and if so, what the answer is. (Even if you know, you don't have to tell!)

tests that tell all

These optional tests serve many purposes, but all reveal gender. (Also see pages 16 and 106 to 109 for more about prenatal tests.)

❖ CVS (chorionic villus sampling), which is performed sometime during weeks 10 to 12, reveals the entire genetic makeup of your baby, including sex.

❖ Amniocentesis, done sometime during weeks 15 to 20, also shows your baby's complete genetic makeup.

❖ A mid-pregnancy ultrasound, around weeks 18 to 20, is a time when your baby's genitals may be clearly visible, particularly if you're having a boy.

CVS and amniocentesis are accurate predictors of sex since they are based on analysis of fetal chromosomes. Ultrasounds are less reliable, depending on the baby's position (some tots are shy!) and variations in the digital image, but if you're lucky, you might spy the evidence for yourself.

week 12

you

❖ Your uterus has moved from the pelvic floor to the front of your abdomen, which can ease some of the pressure on your bladder.

❖ A dark vertical line of pigmentation—known as the linea nigra—may appear on your belly. It typically disappears in the first few months after birth.

your baby

❖ He measures about 2½ inches (6.4 cm) from crown to rump and weighs about half an ounce (14 g).

❖ Your baby can now open his mouth and wiggle his fingers and toes.

"If you can hold out for the surprise, everyone says it's wonderful. I always told myself I would do that, but who was I kidding? I'm an expert at removing tape from presents to see what's inside, then resealing them!"

prep work

Before you spill the beans to your boss, it's a good idea to do some homework.

❖ Read your employer's disability policy. Prenatal complications, labor, and postpartum recovery are covered like any other medical disability. The disability period typically lasts six weeks after a vaginal delivery or eight weeks after a cesarean section.

❖ Find out about your workplace's maternity-leave policy, if it has one. If not, you still might be able to negotiate extra time off or a more flexible schedule upon your return. Also look into applying vacation or sick days to your leave.

❖ If your employer has more than fifty employees, you may be eligible for twelve weeks of leave (but it may be unpaid) under the federal Family and Medical Leave Act.

❖ When you meet with your boss, be ready with an estimated last day at work and return date. Also think about anything you'd like to negotiate, such as returning to work part-time.

thoughts on leaving

If you've been working while simultaneously experiencing the nausea and exhaustion that tends to come with early pregnancy, you may have already started thinking about taking pregnancy and/or maternity leave. Before you talk to your employer about your pregnancy, think about what you want to do and discuss the options with your partner.

On the personal side, you may feel strongly about working up until your due date and returning soon after; or you might find yourself fantasizing about taking pre- and post-birth breaks. Maybe you'd like to downshift to part-time, telecommute, or stop working altogether. Keep in mind that whatever you think now may change when you are closer to your due date and again after your baby comes.

On the practical side, consider what effect your decision will have on your family's finances and what adjustments you might want to start making to your spending and saving habits.

week 13

you

❖ If you poke your belly, your baby will respond with her own movement, but you can't feel it yet.

❖ First-trimester fatigue may be starting to fade.

❖ The top of your uterus is expanding up and out in the lower half of your abdomen—you'll be showing soon.

your baby

❖ From crown to rump, she measures up to 3 inches (7.6 cm). She weighs about ¾ ounce (21 g).

❖ Organs and tissues that took shape during the first trimester are rapidly developing, and her tongue and vocal chords are getting ready for that first cry.

mom to mom

"My hubs and I decided that my working from home would be good for us. He travels, and we both wanted me to be free to hang out with him when he is home. I've been working less and less, so that we can spend more time together, and so I'm less stressed. But by doing that, we are definitely taking an income cut."

changing times

You're officially in your second trimester. Though your belly may still not have officially "popped," you're likely looking rounder. The hormone *relaxin* has loosened ab muscles (making you pooch out) and your joints (making your hips slightly wider).

How are you feeling when you face the new you in the mirror? Some moms-to-be find that they love their rounder, pregnant bodies. Others feel less enthusiastic about changes, for instance, gaining weight in unexpected places, like the arms or neck.

Try to take the changes that come with gaining weight in stride—it's all about nourishing your growing baby.

let it glow

On the bright side, pregnancy hormones sometimes have some pretty sweet effects on your looks.

❖ Great skin: If you're lucky, increased blood flow and changes in oil production are making your skin glow. (Though, for some, increased acne or dryness may result. See page 12 for safe skin-care tips.)

❖ Lusher locks: Normally hair grows, rests, and then falls out. During pregnancy, the falling-out part all but halts, leaving you with thicker hair. The changes in oil production at the follicles may cause wavy hair to curl more, or curly hair to straighten.

❖ Strong nails: They'll probably grow faster and be less likely to chip and break. Hormones play a role in this, but so do your prenatal vitamins. (If you find your nails are dry and cracking, skip polish and moisturize instead.)

take two

The start of your second trimester is a good time to take stock of the perks of pregnancy—hey, no more menstrual cramps! Plus your long-term health outlook improves, too. Pregnancy may decrease your risk of breast and ovarian cancer if you're under 30, and expecting moms often adopt healthier habits (eliminating alcohol, eating better, and quitting smoking) that continue even after the baby's born.

four eyes

Contacts feel like they don't fit anymore? Life looking a little blurrier? Blame it on increased estrogen and see your eye doctor to evaluate your prescription. Dry eyes and light sensitivity are also common. Keep sunglasses and moisturizing eyedrops handy; do not use drops for reducing redness.

week 14

you

❖ You've made it through the first trimester! Nausea now abates for most women.

❖ You may feel sharp aches in your lower abdomen that are the result of ligaments being stretched by your growing uterus (see page 28 for relief tips).

your baby

❖ He measures 3 to 4 inches (7.6 to 10 cm) from crown to rump and weighs about 1½ ounces (43 g).

❖ Genetically determined ridges, visible on his fingertips and palms, will later become his unique handprint.

"I actually felt more confident and beautiful with my big belly than I had ever felt trying to 'compete' in the world of perfect size 4s. For the first time, all of the laws of fashion and beauty didn't apply to me, and the gorgeous swell of my belly made me feel like a goddess!"

dressing the part

Clothes getting uncomfortably snug? Pregnancy provides a great excuse to go shopping! Fortunately, maternity clothes are more stylish and flattering than ever. Here are some shopping tips and ways to get extra mileage out of your current wardrobe:

❖ A buttonhole extender, found at fabric stores, or even a rubber band, gives your fave jeans, pants, and skirts more life; wear 'em unbuttoned with a longer top. Elasticized belly bands serve the same purpose.

❖ Give "regular" size empire-waist tops, sweaters, or tunics a try.

❖ When shopping for maternity tops, look for ones that fit well in the shoulders—these will be most flattering.

❖ Whatever you do, buy what fits—aim for comfortable without being oversized—and don't worry about what size the tag says.

❖ Focus on a few versatile essentials. Three basic black pieces— a dress, pants, and a top—in stretch fabric can be alternated and accessorized in a million ways.

❖ If you work at a job that requires suits or other industry-specific clothing, look for ensembles with mix-and-match pieces.

❖ Avoid buying too far ahead of your growing belly. You may find, for example, that you don't like the feel of pants that sit up high on your belly.

❖ Remember, too, that you'll get use out of maternity togs postpartum, as your body recovers (see page 131).

busted

How quickly you outgrow bras depends on your pre-pregnancy size and how much weight you gain. For now, you might get away with using a bra extender, a small elastic strap that hooks onto your bra to lengthen the rib measurement (available at maternity and fabric stores). Later, you may need progressively bigger and more supportive bras. Let comfort be your guide!

secondhand strategies

Why buy it all new? Raid recently pregnant pals' closets for barely worn maternity gear. You can also buy cute stuff secondhand, at used clothing stores or online.

week 15

you

- ❖ Breathless? During pregnancy you're breathing more frequently and more deeply.

- ❖ Vavoom! If it didn't happen already, you may now be more in the mood for sex. (See page 18.)

- ❖ Sometime during weeks 15 to 20, you may have an amniocentesis performed. (See page 108.)

your baby

- ❖ She measures about 4½ inches (11 cm) from crown to rump and weighs around 2½ ounces (71 g).

- ❖ Hair is sprouting on her head, and she's growing eyebrows. A fine downy hair, known as *lanugo*, covers her body now; it generally disappears before birth or soon after.

mom
to
mom

"You can get different waistbands on maternity pants and skirts: under the belly, over the belly, and mid-belly, or use belly bands on your old clothes. My suggestion—try them all on. Walk around the store. Sit down. Bend over. Get a feel for each kind and then decide what works best for you."

connecting online

At any time in your pregnancy, other moms-to-be and parents can be a great resource—in person or online. Check out local parenting groups with e-mail lists or online postings to get a feel for how they work, and weed out ones that aren't up your alley.

Online forums provide a venue for connecting with others, sharing advice, or commiserating over symptoms, day or night, and continue to be a virtual lifeline after your baby's born. Go to Parenting.com to find bulletin boards for loads of pregnancy issues and new-baby care. But surf with caution.

❖ Don't take everything online as gospel. Many sites have incorrect information, and other parents may have odd ideas or ones that are simply not right.

❖ Watch your online time! It's easy to get sucked into the virtual world, to the detriment of the real one. When you have spare time, ask yourself if you'd rather be surfing or sleeping.

achy abs

If you experience an ache in your lower abdomen (either a quick, sharp pain or a lasting, dull one) it may be round ligament pain. Check with your doctor. Unfortunately, there's not a lot you can do to relieve round ligament pain.

Try lying down on your left side with a pillow under your belly, resting with your knees curled up toward your belly, or taking a warm bath. If the pain becomes severe or moves to your lower back, check back with your doctor.

show me yours

Is your bump popping or somewhat unobtrusive? The way you carry depends on your baby's shape, structure, and position, and your overall muscle tone. If your doc says your baby's growth is on track, you're fine.

left turn

If you sleep on your back, it's time to try a new position. When you lie flat, your increasingly heavy uterus can press down on vital blood vessels, such as the aorta and vena cava, and make you feel faint. Best position for letting the blood flow: on your left side. (Also see page 38.)

week 16

you

❖ Wonder where the weight gain is going? The placenta is about 6 ounces (170 g); amniotic fluid accounts for around 11 ounces (312 g). Each breast has an extra 12 ounces (340 g) or so. The rest is the baby—and you!

❖ If you feel like you have a permanent head cold, blame an increased blood flow to mucous membranes. Get temporary relief with a hot-mist vaporizer or steamy shower.

your baby

❖ He has grown another ½ inch (1.3 cm) since last week and weighs about 3½ ounces (100 g).

❖ His arms and legs are moving about in a sea of amniotic fluid.

mom to mom

"My doctor told me that you shouldn't try to eat things that you hate (in my case, peanut butter and cheese) just for the baby's sake—you can get the vitamins, minerals, and other necessary nutrients from other sources."

heartburn=hair?

Here's an old wives' tale that's actually true: A study conducted at Johns Hopkins University found that 82 percent of women with moderate to severe heartburn delivered babies with full heads of hair; most women with little or no heartburn had bald babies. Researchers think the hormones responsible for heartburn may also trigger fetal hair growth.

everyone's an expert

Now that your pregnancy is becoming apparent, you can expect unsolicited advice to pour in from every direction—even from strangers on the street. Support, especially from other moms, can be great. But there will be folks who feel compelled to tell you what you should be eating, drinking, naming your baby, and so on.

Some of the advice you may be offered will boil down to old wives' tales: Raising your arms over your head causes the umbilical cord to wrap around your baby's neck (false). Be prepared to hear some well-intended but incorrect information.

How to handle the pregnancy police? Respond with a polite "Interesting," or "We're doing fine, thanks," before changing the subject. You can also simply smile and walk away. Even if the person is speaking from experience, try not to compare yourself to others or expect that your pregnancy will be like anyone else's—every woman's body is unique.

heading off busybodies

There are a lot of different ways to get pregnant, be pregnant, and give birth. And everyone has an opinion on how you should do it. How much you share is up to you, but be prepared to field personal questions.

To handle nosy inquiries—especially from strangers—about, say, whether you had fertility treatments or if you're planning to have an epidural, prepare some stock responses. You might smile and say something vague like, "Thanks for your interest," or "We're keeping it to ourselves." Don't feel guilty about not answering a question directly; you're entitled to your privacy.

When the intrusive question comes from a close relative or friend, you'll probably want to employ a little more finesse. Tactful options include, "This is what works best for us," "My doctor is comfortable with this," and good old "We haven't decided yet."

week 17

you

❖ Your growing uterus is about 2 inches (5 cm) below your belly button, pushing up against and shifting your intestines aside and expanding your belly outward.

❖ If you didn't before, you are starting to look more like a pregnant woman now— and not like someone who has just packed on a couple of pounds.

your baby

❖ From crown to rump she measures 5 to 5½ inches (12.7 to 14 cm) and weighs about 5¼ ounces (150 g).

❖ She's got eyelashes.

❖ Fat is starting to fill out her body and keep her warm. By the time she's born, fat will account for two-thirds of her weight.

mom to mom

"Everyone wants to connect with you and that new life, be it touching your belly or sharing their own stories—some of which are awful! But keep in mind that your experience will be unique—then it's easier to keep perspective, thank them, and tune most of it out."

Scope out places at or near work, such as comfy café chairs or lobby couches, where you can catch a quick nap when midday fatigue hits. You can keep a rolled-up mat and blanket under your desk to pull out when the coast is clear.

letting go

Need an easy way to relax? Try progressive relaxation: Sit or lie in a comfortable position. Starting with your toes and working your way up toward your head, tense and then release muscles in each part of your body. Breathe deeply and focus on one area at a time.

get out of town!

Got the urge for a pre-baby vacation? The second trimester's combo of increased energy and not-yet-cumbersome belly makes travel easier.

❖ When flying, opt for the aisle seat so you can get up and walk around easily. That helps you avoid leg cramps and swollen ankles, and reduces your risk of dangerous blood clots that pregnant women are more prone to.

❖ On the road: Plan frequent stops to stretch your legs and use the bathroom. And be sure to wear your seat belt: Tuck the bottom strap under your bump.

❖ Pack your own healthy snacks to avoid vending machines and dubious airport options. Tote plenty of water or, if flying, a container to fill after you go through airport security.

❖ Don't plan to travel after week 36. If your pregnancy is high risk, your doctor may restrict travel sooner.

worry busters

Can you be a mom and not worry? Probably impossible! Most moms-to-be feel more carefree in their second trimester, with things humming along nicely. Still, you might find plenty to obsess over, from your baby's health to your ability to be a good mom. Hormone-induced mood swings may make stress worse.

Information is your best defense against needless worry. Talk to your doctor and veteran moms about any health-related fears. And let go of the notion of the "perfect mother." She doesn't exist.

Don't deny the power of distraction! Clear your mind with a juicy book, a favorite CD, lunch with a friend, or an escapist movie. Or try proven relaxation tools, such as meditation, yoga, or massage. Often, relief comes as your baby more fully develops and you can feel her kick. However, if you experience extreme or ongoing anxiety, talk to your doctor.

week 18

you

- Your uterus is about the size of a cantaloupe.

- The hormone relaxin is causing your joints to loosen, especially in your lower back and hips. See page 36 for safe stretching tips.

- Sometime in the next few weeks, you may have a mid-pregnancy ultrasound.

your baby

- Go ahead and sing to your baby—outside sounds filter through the bones forming in his ear.

- His retinas are more sensitive to light now; he'll perceive a red glow when you're in the sunlight.

- Swallowing, sucking, and making faces are all part of your baby's repertoire.

"Looking at my ultrasound pictures always made me smile. No matter how awful I felt or how up-and-down my emotions were, seeing that little baby taking shape just made me feel giddy!"

the weight-gain train

As you hit the halfway point, note your weight gain so far. You'll likely have added between 8 and 14 pounds, unless your doc has given you other advice that's specific to your situation. Under or over the mark? Evaluate what you've been eating.

Gaining too much too fast increases your risk of complications, like high blood pressure. But don't go too far the other way; a restrictive diet deprives your baby of essential nutrients.

Try to hit the diet sweet spot by focusing on foods that pack a nutritional punch. Fill your plate with fresh fruits and vegetables. Pick whole grains (brown rice, whole-wheat bread, and whole-grain pasta) over refined (white rice, bread, and pasta) and low-fat dairy over higher-fat options. Amp up your calcium intake with daily servings of low-fat yogurt, milk, or hard cheese. Drink a smoothie made with low-fat frozen yogurt, skim milk, and fruit to get an all-in-one serving of protein, calcium, vitamins, and fiber.

stark raving craving

Move over pickles! In the United States, citrus fruits are among the most popular pregnancy food cravings. Next on the list is ice cream—naturally! Pizza, pasta, hamburgers, and Mexican food are close runners-up. Here are some healthy ways to sate your cravings:

❖ Opt for lower-fat versions of desired snacks, such as low-fat ice cream or frozen yogurt.

❖ Got a sweet tooth? Try dried fruit. Or have a small serving of high-quality dark chocolate or a mini-size candy bar.

❖ In place of donuts, reach for fruit breads or low-fat muffins.

❖ Swap out sugary sodas for 100-percent fruit juices diluted with water, or water with lemon or lime slices.

❖ To feed a salt craving, pick pickles or pretzels instead of chips.

❖ When eating out: Try vegetables instead of pepperoni or sausage on pizza, a turkey or veggie patty rather than beef for your burger, steamed rice instead of fried at a Chinese place, or whole beans in place of refried at a Mexican cantina.

it's okay to worry

Pregnancy can bring out your inner worrywart. Are you gaining the right amount of weight? Is your baby healthy? Will you be a good mom? Why did you do this in the first place?!? Pregnancy hormones and poor sleep magnify your worries. Most of what you're feeling is normal, but talk to your doctor if anxiety is getting the better of you.

ease the burn

Suffering from heartburn? Eating slowly and having small, more-frequent meals may help. Other relief strategies: Skip fatty, acidic, or spicy foods; wait a few hours after eating before lying down; or try sipping flat ginger ale or eating yogurt. Talk to your doctor before taking antacids.

week 19

you

- A combination of gravity and blood pressure dips can make you feel dizzy when you stand up too fast. Get in the habit of rising slowly.

- Feel butterflies in your stomach? Called *quickening*, that may be your first inkling of your baby's movements. Some women don't feel a thing until around week 24.

your baby

- She measures 6½ inches (16.5 cm) from crown to rump and weighs about 9 ounces (255 g).

- Motor neurons between the muscles and brain are connecting, allowing your mini-gymnast to roll, kick, and stretch at will.

"During my first pregnancy, I moved to California where I craved New York City pretzels so badly that my grandmother wrapped six in tin foil and mailed them to me. I was so thankful!"

get up and go

Take advantage of increased energy to stick with or improve exercise habits. If nausea kept you on the bench for the first trimester, start slowly and get the green light from your health-care provider first, especially if your pregnancy is considered high risk. If you've been working out all along, keep up the good work! Exercise builds strength, increases endurance, and boosts energy. More good news: Research shows that being in shape physically can lead to shorter labor, reduce your risk of birth complications, and speed postpartum recovery.

rules of the game

Whether you're new to exercise, or you're a regular fitness junkie, here are a few pregnancy-specific precautions (also see page 14).

❖ Loose joints and the additional weight they're now supporting mean that high-impact exercise is out. You can still jog, walk, take low-impact exercise classes, do strength training, and ride a stationary bike. No-impact options, like water aerobics or swimming, are also great prenatal exercise.

❖ If you're looking to add some gentle exercise or to replace a more strenuous routine, prenatal yoga can improve your strength and stamina, and give you an opportunity to practice deep-breathing techniques that you can use during labor.

❖ Skip routines that call for you to lie flat on your back—or belly!

❖ Sit-ups and crunches are out. These may cause your rectus muscles to separate (along the line that runs down the center of your "six-pack"), which can cause back problems. (See page 58 for a safe ab exercise.)

❖ Listen to your body. Slow down or rest if you find yourself panting or feel overheated.

safe stretching

Limber is the name of the game in pregnancy—relaxin gets your body ready for birth by making joints and ligaments loosey-goosey.

Your newly stretchy status can leave you injury prone, though, so be gentle with your joints. Breathe deeply while you relax your muscles, and try to ease into a stretch—never force it! Avoid arching your back or hyperextending or bending any joints too far.

snack attack

About an hour before you exercise, eat a light snack. A piece of fruit or whole-grain crackers—combined with a protein such as hard cheese or nuts—will help keep you from getting light-headed.

week 20

you

❖ Your uterus is growing at the pace of about ½ inch (1 cm) each week. Expect questions from strangers about when you're due.

❖ The growing weight of your belly shifts your posture and can cause lower back pain, so if you sit a lot, get up frequently to move around and stretch.

your baby

❖ He measures 7 inches (18 cm) from crown to rump and weighs about 11 ounces (312 g).

❖ A creamy protective coating called the *vernix caseosa* covers his skin.

❖ Your baby's lungs can't breathe air yet, but his chest is moving up and down. Think of it as practice!

mom to mom

"I walked, swam, did yoga, and stretched. Everything I did was easily accessible and inexpensive. The walking was free, my condo had a pool, I took a yoga class at a nearby community center for very little money, and I stretched at home. I kept it simple, easy, and enjoyable."

back to school

Now is a good time to sign up for any pregnancy- and parenting-related classes that you want to take during your third trimester, since prenatal workshops tend to fill up quickly (see page 116).

Most hospitals offer a basic childbirth preparation course over one to three days. Other more in-depth classes that cover "natural" (meaning nonmedical) pain management and partner-assisted birth techniques can run anywhere from four to twelve weeks. Research your options and ask for recommendations from other parents before signing up.

Unless you've already had experience with babies, you may want to take a baby-care class, which usually covers the basics of changing diapers, dressing, and bathing. (Most hospital nurses will also give you a refresher on this before you take your baby home.) Also consider signing up for a class on infant first aid and CPR. And definitely consider taking a breastfeeding class: Even though it's "natural," breastfeeding can be plenty tricky to master (see page 130), and a class can help you learn what to expect.

Hospitals usually offer workshops, too, as do birthing centers and community organizations devoted to new-parent education. You can also ask your health-care provider to recommend classes. And don't forget to check out the baby-care videos on Parenting.com.

birth 101

While the content of childbirth classes will vary, you can expect yours to cover these basic topics:

❖ The stages of labor and delivery (see pages 114 to 115)

❖ Pain-relief methods, including breathing and relaxation techniques, birthing positions, and medical options

❖ Possible medical interventions, including c-sections

❖ Your partner's role during labor and delivery

❖ Postpartum topics such as breastfeeding and circumcision

take a breather

Try this fast energy booster: Sit in a chair with your legs parted. Take a deep breath. As you let it out, gently drop your head toward your knees and reach for your toes. Don't overstretch. Rest here for a bit, then breathe in. Slowly straighten up. Repeat as many times as you like.

read all about it

Think you're having sleep troubles now? Just wait: Sleep deprivation goes along with being a new parent. Consider reading up on the topic of sleep now. You'll gain insight into your sleep habits and a head start on ideas for helping your baby sleep.

week 21

you

❖ The top of your uterus has risen to about ½ inch (1 cm) above your navel.

❖ You're probably feeling pretty good now, thanks to an ongoing second-trimester energy boost.

your baby

❖ Length is now measured from head to toe, and she's about 10½ inches (27 cm) long. She weighs more than 12½ ounces (354 g).

❖ Your baby now swallows amniotic fluid—which provides up to 15 percent of her nutritional needs and helps prepare her body for eating and digesting once she's born.

❖ She recognizes flavor, too: Taste buds have developed on her tongue.

mom to mom

"I went shopping for bedding with my husband, now that we know we're having a girl. I pointed to a set I liked, and my husband's face lit up. He announced, 'That's perfect for my Princess!' Our little girl already has him wrapped around her finger, and she hasn't even made an appearance!"

all dressed up

Sweet little baby outfits with matching hats are hard to resist (and they're popular baby gifts). What your baby needs most, though, in the early months are washable basic layette items: lots of snap-bottom bodysuits and one-piece footed outfits and sleepers (see page 90). Keep tags on clothes and hang on to gift receipts until you know the size and season match up, in case you need to make an exchange.

cry busters

Guaranteed: Your newborn will cry at least some of the time. Advice: Have different soothing gear at the ready: swaddling blankets (see page 81), pacifiers (if you plan to use them), a bouncy seat, and a sling or front carrier (see page 86).

getting in gear

Shopaholics rejoice—now is a good time to start gathering or registering for the baby gear you'll want on hand for your newborn's arrival. (See pages 90 to 91 for a detailed checklist.)

That said, don't go crazy just yet. The list of what you truly need in the first months with your newborn is surprisingly small:

❖ A place for your baby to sleep (see page 80)

❖ Diapers, wipes, a changing pad, and diaper cream (see page 82)

❖ A car seat to take baby home from the hospital (see page 84)

❖ A stroller (see page 86)

❖ Layette: Clothes (see "all dressed up," left), burp cloths, and receiving or swaddling blankets

❖ Medical supplies: a rectal thermometer and a nasal aspirator to suck mucus out of a congested nose (see page 91)

❖ What can wait: a highchair, childproofing gear, most baby toys

showering your baby

Many lucky moms-to-be are treated to a baby shower. Whether it's a surprise or the hostess consults you in advance, consider it an opportunity to be showered in good wishes (and, yes, gifts).

Showers are often scheduled in the last trimester, but shouldn't be held too close to your due date—you may be too uncomfortable or even go into labor early. Have a January due date? It's smart to have the shower before holiday happenings fill up everyone's calendar. Or hold off until after the baby's born; some moms-to-be do so for religious or personal reasons.

If you're asked for a list of invitees, include address, phone, and e-mail. And send thank-you notes as promptly as possible. After the baby arrives, you'll have to start all over again!

week 22

you

- Don't be surprised if you're still sensitive to certain scents you used to love, from bacon to coffee to your favorite perfume.

- You've probably felt your baby move by now—get ready for the activity to really pick up!

your baby

- He measures about 11 inches (28 cm) from head to toe and weighs about 1 pound (454 g).

- He now registers the sensation of touch as he rolls, kicks, and stretches inside of you.

- His teeth are starting to develop below the gum line.

"If you're having a shower and are telling people whether you're having a boy or girl, be sure of the sex. Mistakes are not that uncommon. My dad and stepmom thought my sister was a boy for two months, until the doctor said, 'Oops.'"

dream decorating

When decorating a nursery, a good first step is to pick a theme, style, or color scheme. While the traditional pink, blue, or unisex yellow or green will always remain popular, you can also choose from a variety of contemporary palettes ranging from bold saturated colors to quiet neutrals.

A growing trend is to decorate a nursery in the same style as the rest of the home. Whether sleek modern or shabby chic, this approach simplifies choices, since you already have a starting point, and tends to age better than an infant-oriented theme.

But if a baby theme inspires you, go for it. Trains, ducks, flowers, ABCs . . . your choices are endless. Artsy types can turn a room into a spaceship, a castle, or the ocean deep. Also think about graphic themes, such as stripes, gingham, or stars. Just think: It'll be quite a while before your baby has an opinion, so it's all up to you! (See page 80 for more on setting up the nursery.)

going green

Looking for organic and eco-friendly options for the nursery?

❖ Untreated solid wood furniture, made of sustainably harvested birch or maple, is nice, but pricey. Cribs made of painted metal are a cheaper earth-friendly option.

❖ Low- or zero-VOC (volatile organic compound) paint helps keep the air clear of toxic fumes.

❖ Organic mattresses are expensive but worth springing for, since your baby's face will come closest to the materials in them for a large part of her nights and days. (If you buy a conventional crib mattress, air it out for at least a month before using it.)

❖ Sheets labeled "flame retardant" or "water resistant" are treated with chemicals. Opt for organic or all-cotton bed linens instead.

stylist's tip

Because it's far easier to match paint to prints than the other way around, pick patterned items first—rugs, bedding, artwork, window treatments. Then choose a paint color. Have someone else paint. It's not good for you to climb ladders and breathe fumes.

nursery basics

If you want specific nursery furniture by the time the baby arrives, order soon, because large items such as cribs, dressers, and changing tables often take months to arrive. But don't stress over it. All you really need at first is a spot for her to sleep (see page 80). You can feed her in bed or any comfortable chair, and lay a changing pad on the floor for diapering.

week 23

you

❖ As your uterus continues to inch upward and your shape rounds, your belly button may turn from an innie to an outie.

❖ Your appetite may be raging—nature's way of encouraging you to meet your baby's nutrient needs.

your baby

❖ She measures about 11½ inches (29 cm) from head to toe and weighs about 1¼ pounds (567 g).

❖ Her movements are more sophisticated. For instance, she can stretch her arms and trail her hands along the umbilical cord.

❖ Her hearing is so clear that loud noises can startle her, making her heart thump and arms flail. She much prefers soft music—and the sound of your voice.

mom to mom

"Every time I felt overwhelmed, I would go into the unfinished nursery and do something productive like put together a bookcase or fill up the diaper hanger. Just being in the nursery brought me instant calm. And a small powdered doughnut didn't hurt either."

sleep like a baby

If you're having trouble sleeping already, you're not alone. And when others make jokes about a poor night's sleep being "good practice," you may not find it so funny. Adjust your nighttime routine to pack in good ZZZs:

❖ If your bed doesn't provide enough support, invest in a dense mattress pad that also has some give—the foam kind, shaped like an egg carton, is an inexpensive option.

❖ A body pillow can make side sleeping easier and cozier. Or place extra pillows wherever they may increase comfort: behind your back, under the side of your belly, between your knees, and even between your breasts.

❖ Try to regulate sleep-and-wake times to "train" your body to sleep consistent hours.

❖ Are middle-of-the-night bathroom breaks wearing you out? Consume most of your liquid intake during the day and then taper off at night. Go to the bathroom right before lights out.

❖ Night sweats? To cool down, wear light cotton pajamas, and keep an extra pair near your bed in case you have to change out of sweaty ones during the night. Make sure to replenish those fluids by drinking plenty of water during the day.

❖ Soothing smells can work wonders to lure you back to sleep. Try a lavender-scented pillow or eye mask.

dreams may come

It's common during pregnancy to have comforting, fascinating, or even disturbing or frightening dreams. Go ahead and blame your hormones, which play havoc with sleep patterns. Add in natural fears about childbirth and motherhood, and you may be in for a dream-packed night.

If your dreams are stressing you out, don't keep it to yourself. It helps to talk it out. Talk to your partner, who may also be having some baby-related nightmares, or friends who have been there. (See week 18 for more tips on easing anxiety.)

week 24

you

❖ Your uterus has risen to 2 inches (5 cm) above your belly button.

❖ Between weeks 24 and 28, expect to have a glucose screening test to assess the risk of gestational diabetes. (See page 107.)

your baby

❖ Your baby is about 12 inches (30 cm) from head to toe and weighs over 1⅓ pounds (600 g).

❖ He's so active, it probably feels like he's turning cartwheels and somersaults in there, especially when you attempt to go to sleep.

❖ His face is complete: Eyes, ears, nose, and mouth are just where they should be.

mom
to
mom

"The first few weeks of bed rest are the hardest, trying to adjust mentally to the new routine. After you adjust, it will be bearable. You just have to make the most of it. Movies, books, puzzles, and writing letters all helped me. So did inviting friends over once a week for dinner—ordering in, of course."

a little romance

Last chance alert: Consider a "babymoon," or quick romantic getaway with your partner, before your baby arrives. (For tips on safety and comfort while flying or road-tripping, see page 32.)

❖ Search online or talk to travel agents who may know about special babymoon packages that include spa treatments, candlelight dinners, and the like.

❖ Keep in mind, the longer you wait, the bigger you'll be, and the more awkward you may feel, which may affect how far from home you'll want to travel.

❖ Your getaway doesn't have to be a long, complicated vacation. Consider a road trip to a nearby bed-and-breakfast, a weekend at a beach resort, or a dinner and overnight stay at a hotel.

skin soothers

Stretching skin leaving you dry and itchy? Hydrate, hydrate, hydrate. In addition to drinking lots of water, bathe in warm (not hot) water, use gentle, non-soap cleanser, and pile on lotion or oil while your skin is still damp.

Are stretch marks showing up? There's no proof that the various lotions and potions prevent or cure them; the condition is genetic. But if you want to, pick a product that smells and feels nice, or just grab some olive, almond, or coconut oil, and rub it on.

To help prickly heat rash, which may show up in the folds of your skin or around your bra and panty lines, wear breathable, natural fabrics, such as cotton, to ventilate skin and aid healing.

Wearing the "mask of pregnancy" (aka *chloasma* or *melasma*)? Hormones and sun exposure cause these dark splotches, usually on the cheeks, upper lip, and forehead. They should subside after birth. For now, apply broad-spectrum sunscreen (SPF 30 or higher) and hold off on treatment: Don't use bleaching agents.

Moles and birthmarks may darken a bit, and new moles may appear, all of which is normal—unless you notice a change in the shape or size of a specific mole or mark, or it starts to itch. In that case, see a dermatologist right away to have it checked.

in the mood

As your belly grows, you may want to try different sexual positions—you on top, spooning, or doggy style—to find the most comfortable ones for you and your partner.

fluid situation

Puffy feet and ankles? It's edema, caused by water retention and made worse in hot and humid weather. Drink plenty of water, avoid crossing your legs while sitting, and prop your feet up whenever possible. Stay cool and wear light layers. Normally, edema is more annoying than worrisome. Call your doctor if swelling comes on suddenly, or your hands and face puff up unusually; these can be signs of preeclampsia—pregnancy-induced hypertension.

week 25

you

❖ Your uterus has reached the size of a soccer ball.

❖ Your belly may visibly move now as your baby moves.

❖ Stretch marks—discolored linear patterns on the skin—may appear across your abdomen, as well as on your hips and breasts.

your baby

❖ She measures about 13½ inches (34 cm) from head to toe and weighs 1½ pounds (680 g).

❖ She can make a fist and touch her toes.

❖ Her heartbeat can now be heard by an ear pressed up against your belly.

"When I was pregnant, my skin itched so much! I washed and moisturized my belly twice a day. If your doctor gives you the okay, look into oatmeal baths for soothing really itchy skin."

47

balancing act

As your belly grows, your center of gravity starts to shift forward, leaving you off balance and at greater risk of taking a tumble. To stay on an even keel, slow *waaaay* down. Wear shoes with traction, use handrails on stairs, and be especially careful when walking on slippery surfaces. As much as possible, have others do the picking up. Even lifting a pet can cause you to lose your balance.

kick me

This week your doctor may ask you to start counting kicks. Keep in mind that the most important number is your own daily count—comparing your baby to herself, not to other babies. As a general rule, if you don't feel ten movements in two hours, call your health-care provider.

put labor off

Few possibilities frighten an expectant mother more than preterm labor (defined as labor starting before week 37). If you experience any of these symptoms, call your doctor right away: consistent contractions (every 10 minutes), abdominal or pelvic pressure, mild cramping, unusual vaginal discharge, or lower back pain.

There is no known cause of preterm labor, but experts believe certain factors increase a woman's risk, including: smoking, high blood pressure, diabetes, carrying multiples, uterine infection during pregnancy, being 35 or older, preeclampsia, and being over- or underweight. Here's what may help prevent it:

❖ Eat right. Stick to a healthy diet, including sources of omega-3 fatty acids (such as wild salmon), calcium (milk, yogurt), and vitamin C (citrus fruit); and try to maintain a healthy weight gain. (For more food information, see pages 98 to 99.)

❖ Take care of your teeth. Brush with a soft toothbrush, floss regularly, and have routine teeth cleanings to reduce your risk of an infection. (Also see page 12.)

❖ Take medications only with your doctor's approval.

labor warm-up

You might feel your uterus tighten up for a minute or two; this sensation is probably not a sign of preterm labor but rather a Braxton Hicks contraction, or false labor pain. These contractions are normal and help the body prepare for delivery. Monitor the frequency and let your doctor know about them, especially if they become regular or painful. (For a more detailed comparison of false and true labor, see page 62.)

week 26

you

❖ You're almost two-thirds of the way through your pregnancy—and you're feeling it! Backache and pressure in your pelvic area are common.

❖ If you're one of the lucky ones, you're sporting a luxuriously full mane of pregnancy hair by now (see page 24).

your baby

❖ He measures 14 inches (35.5 cm) from head to toe and weighs just under 2 pounds (907 g).

❖ Your baby is growing faster, and his brain is maturing rapidly.

❖ Almost fully developed and nearly ready to open, his eyes are blue now. The color may change, depending on his genetics.

 mom to mom

"My husband says the baby is awake when he gets up for work in the morning. He will lay in bed with his hands on my belly for about 15 minutes. I am fast asleep, but he says that is when she does her morning aerobics."

the name game

Three months left: It may seem like an awfully long time, but will it be enough to settle on a name for your baby? Time to start mulling if you haven't already! Are there names you've always liked? Is there a family member you want to honor? Guessing who this little person will be, what he or she may grow up to be like—even what you want to call out to your child when it's time for dinner—can be an exciting and daunting project.

Keep a running list on page 140, jotting down every name that comes to mind—don't censor yourself just yet. Even if you feel set on a name, you still might want to keep brainstorming. Visit Parenting.com/babynames for some suggestions. If you get overwhelmed, put your list aside. Sometimes the obvious choice comes to you in the delivery room!

No doubt people will pester you for your faves. Share if you like, but be aware that doing so leaves you open for less-than-positive reactions. Maybe it's best to keep the candidates secret for now!

plan for the memories

Take the time now to gather up gear that will help you record all of those special memories to come.

❖ If you don't already own an easy-to-use camera, shop around for one to bring to the hospital.

❖ Take the time now to learn how to use new equipment. Practice by having your partner photograph your bump.

❖ Be sure to buy extra batteries and memory cards.

❖ Crafty moms-to-be may want to pick up a baby journal, hand- or footprint kits, scrapbooking supplies, or picture frames.

❖ If you want to use an online photo-sharing service, set up an account and send your friends and relatives the username and password. Or if you're setting up a website, send out the URL.

week 27

_____

_____

_____

_____

_____

_____

_____

_____

_____

_____

you

❖ You may start to feel winded even more quickly, as your growing uterus crowds your diaphragm.

❖ Got leg cramps? Flex your feet, especially before you go to bed, massage your legs, stay hydrated, and take regular walks to get relief. Avoid pointing your toes.

your baby

❖ She measures about 14½ inches (37 cm) from head to toe and weighs just over 2 pounds (907 g).

❖ Thumb sucking is a new favorite activity—and good practice. This helps your baby self-soothe in the early months, and it strengthens her cheeks and jaw.

❖ Your bambina is bulking up with layers of fat to keep herself warm. Her immune system is gearing up, too.

mom to mom

"My husband and I found out our baby's gender both times, but we didn't announce their names. We gave them 'prenatal names' so we could keep our choices private. Leah's was 'Mavis,' and Ben's was 'Melvin.' It was fun to see people's faces when they thought those were their real names!"

put the squeeze on

Prepare for the labor of labor—and reduce the risk of postpartum incontinence—with Kegels, an exercise designed to strengthen the muscles of the pelvic floor.

To do a Kegel, squeeze the muscles that you use to stop the flow of urine. Hold for 10 seconds, then release. Rest for 10 seconds. Repeat. Too long? Start with 3 to 5 seconds and increase the duration as you get stronger. Try to repeat the contraction ten times in a row, ideally three times a day.

To make Kegels less like a chore, work them into your day during a phone call or meeting, while watching a movie, or before you go to sleep. Try them during sex—they may increase stimulation of your clitoris, which can enhance enjoyment.

As you get closer to your due date, try to add more Kegel reps to your daily regimen. If you can, add five contractions per set each week, until you're doing thirty at a time. Don't stress, though, about the exact number you do—some are better than none!

take a tour

You don't want to arrive at the hospital, in the throes of labor, and not know where to go or how to check in! Most hospitals offer tours, so take advantage. Ask questions and take notes!

❖ What registration forms can you fill out in advance?

❖ What type of ID will be required?

❖ Where is the maternity entrance and check-in area?

❖ Are there any special parking procedures?

❖ How many visitors are allowed in the labor/delivery and postpartum rooms? What are visiting hours?

❖ Are postpartum rooms private or shared?

❖ What are the procedures for anesthesiologists/epidurals?

❖ Are there lactation consultants on staff?

❖ Where can your partner sleep?

week 28

you

- ❖ Ideally, you've gained between 17 and 24 pounds (8 to 11 kg) by now, unless otherwise advised by your doctor (see page 10).

- ❖ Be easy on yourself. Due to fluctuating hormone levels, you may be experiencing mood swings. Writing about your emotions could help.

your baby

- ❖ He measures approximately 15 inches (38 cm) from head to toe and weighs close to 2¼ pounds (1 kg).

- ❖ Brain tissue is developing folds and grooves on what was once a smooth surface.

- ❖ His eyes have opened— he'll use his hands to shield them if light shines in his direction.

 mom to mom

"I was giving my husband a hug, and he pulled up my shirt a bit to rub my belly. When I moved, my bellybutton popped out a bit and then went back in—we were cracking up, it looked so strange! When my belly gets bigger, I'm going to end up with an 'outie' that looks like the popper on a turkey."

team labor

While your partner is probably planning to be at your side during labor offering encouragement and back rubs, a family member, a close friend, or a professional labor coach (called a doula) can provide support for both of you. This person can help distract you during those long hours; give your partner bathroom, meal, and sleep breaks; and run interference, keeping friends or relatives at bay until you're ready to see them.

Doulas receive special training in the physiology of birth, as well as in how to support and advocate for a laboring woman. If you hire a doula, she'll coach you through your labor from the first contraction to your baby's first cry (see DONA.org).

so-so on sex?

Sex drive may rise and fall like a roller coaster all throughout your pregnancy. The third trimester brings some other concerns into the bedroom.

❖ There may be a mismatch between desire and, um, ability. Though you may be in the mood (in part thanks to increased blood flow to your vaginal area), you may be so generally uncomfortable that you don't even feel like attempting the act. It's okay (and common) to opt out for now (see page 18).

❖ If you're concerned about hurting the baby, don't let that cool your jets. He's well cushioned in the womb, and your cervix is shut tight.

❖ Worried about lying flat on your back? While you don't want to spend too much time prone, it's okay for short periods, as long as your partner's supporting his own weight. Or try other positions, including you on top, spooning, or doggy style.

❖ Many women feel post-sex contractions, but they're usually nothing to be concerned about. However, let your doctor know if contractions become strong and regular, or if you have any spotting or bleeding. (See page 62 for labor signs.)

week 29

_____

_____

_____

_____

_____

_____

_____

_____

_____

_____

_____

_____

you

❖ Your uterus has risen to about 4 inches (10 cm) above the navel.

❖ Your growing breasts may need yet another larger bra.

your baby

❖ She's about 15½ inches (39 cm) from head to toe and 2¾ pounds (1.2 kg). She now looks more like a real baby than a developing fetus.

❖ Vigorous kicks and jabs may make it seem like she's moving all day long.

❖ She may already be in the head-down position in preparation for birth, but if she's not, there's still plenty of time for her to turn.

mom to mom

"My husband thought having sex while I was pregnant was weird and swore he would poke our son in the head. Ridiculous, I know. He was also terrified that he would accidentally break my water, leaving himself traumatized for life. I had to practically force him to have sex!"

child watch

Who will watch your baby if you return to work or simply need extra help? Your decision will depend on factors such as location, the hours of care you need, and the cost. Here are some tips on finding a good match:

- ❖ Do you prefer a nanny, au pair, home-based day care, a larger facility, or an occasional sitter? Be open-minded: You might start out looking at centers and discover a home-based day care that's perfect for you.

- ❖ Start looking now. Some providers have waiting lists and spots often fill up months in advance, especially for infants.

- ❖ Set a realistic budget. You want the best care possible, while not eating up your entire check to pay the sitter!

- ❖ Good referral sources include word of mouth, parenting groups, and colleges. You can also connect with potential candidates online. Try SitterCity.com or Care.com.

- ❖ Child-care service agencies do the legwork and background checks, but you will pay a hefty fee.

- ❖ Start with a telephone interview. If you like what you hear, schedule a visit.

see for yourself

Before you choose your child-care provider, observe the person or staff in action with children. If you find a center you like, make a second unannounced visit, preferably during drop-off or pick-up times, which tend to be the most hectic. That way you can see how parents and caregivers interact, and how relaxed (or not!) everyone is. Always check references before hiring.

paying for child care

If your employer offers a Flexible Spending Account (FSA), to put aside pretax dollars to pay for child care, get the forms now. Even if you're on leave, you still have only thirty days after birth to sign up.

ask away

Narrow down your top day-care providers by asking lots of questions:

- ❖ What is your training in child development, infant CPR, and first aid?

- ❖ What's your work history?

- ❖ What's your technique for calming a crying baby? Getting him to sleep?

- ❖ How do you envision a typical day?

- ❖ What's the backup plan if you're sick?

week 30

you

❖ You may feel an increased need to go to the bathroom at night as your growing uterus puts the squeeze on your bladder.

❖ Hormones continue to soften the tissues around your joints, making it even easier to overextend them—so be careful when moving around.

your baby

❖ From head to toe, he's about 16 inches (41 cm) long and weighs around 3 pounds (1.4 kg). Babies usually gain up to 8 ounces (227 g) a week from here on out.

❖ When he's not bopping around and nudging you, he is sleeping.

❖ He has the eyelashes and the head of hair (if any) he'll be born with.

"I already have a three-year-old daughter. It's been very interesting trying to explain the whole baby concept to her. She understands that we're going to get a baby sometime, but she thinks that we'll have to buy it from the store."

splitsville

Strong abdominals are a plus when it comes time to push during labor, but it's not safe to do sit-ups or crunches during pregnancy. They put too much pressure on your outer ab muscle, which may have split down the middle by now—a condition called *diastasis recti*. The best strategy: strengthening your transverse ab muscle, which wraps around your belly and back. Try this exercise:

Sit with your shoulders over your hips. Inhale deeply, expanding your belly as you breathe in. Then as you exhale, contract your abs to pull your belly button in, first about halfway back to your spine, and then all the way back. Squeeze and hold; then release to the halfway point; don't go all the way back to the expanded position. Each squeeze and release counts as one contraction. Repeat as many times as you feel comfortable doing, up to a set of twenty-five several times a day. Don't stress about the number—just do them when you think of it. Some are better than none.

back support

The extra weight in front combined with the effects of relaxin on your joints can be a recipe for chronic backaches. Try these tactics to help ease the stress on your body:

❖ Kneel on all fours, back straight, and gently tilt your pelvis forward and back to release tension.

❖ Try a supportive maternity belt to lighten the load.

❖ Sleep on your left side with knees bent. Place a pillow behind your back and one between your knees.

❖ Squat from your knees if you have to lift something up. Better yet, ask someone to get it for you!

❖ Spend some time in a pool to take the weight off your back, hips, and legs.

❖ Chiropractic treatment or a prenatal massage (see page 68) may help your pain subside.

week 31

_____

_____

_____

_____

_____

_____

_____

_____

_____

_____

_____

you

❖ Pressure from your uterus forcing blood and fluids to your legs may cause your feet and ankles to swell (see page 46).

❖ Your growing uterus is squeezing your stomach, too, making it difficult to finish a meal.

your baby

❖ She measures about 16½ inches (42 cm) from head to toe and weighs around 3½ pounds (1.6 kg).

❖ She can blink her eyes.

❖ The fine hair (lanugo) that appeared on her body several weeks ago is disappearing.

mom to mom

"When my back was really painful, I would get on my knees and try to stretch my muscles. That at least took some of the pain away. Unfortunately, I think the pain is one of those rites of passage for mothers, but worth it in the end when you hold your little creation."

59

pediatrician decision

Now is the time to choose your baby's pediatrician, who will examine him in the hospital after delivery. This decision involves a combination of practical considerations and gut feelings.

On the practical side, make a list of doctors who are part of your health insurance network and affiliated with the hospital where you will be delivering; then check which ones are convenient to home, work, or day care. Cross reference that list with word-of-mouth recommendations and the American Board of Pediatrics' website (ABP.org) to check for clean records.

Interview a few likely candidates (see page 110). The "X" factor is all about how you respond to each doctor's demeanor.

money talks

Becoming a parent will alter your spending and saving needs, and possibly your family's income. Before your baby arrives, you might want to take some time to tackle these tasks:

❖ Write a will—or update an existing one—to spell out where your assets would go if something happens to you, your partner, or both of you, and who would take guardianship of your child.

❖ Buy or update life insurance.

❖ Try to reduce debt, such as credit cards or student loans.

❖ If your income will be going down during maternity leave or because you're leaving a job to stay at home, consider setting money aside now.

❖ Research college-savings plans, so that if you want to start taking advantage of tax-saving options, such as 529 plans, starting from day one, you're ready. Consult a financial planner on the best strategy for your family.

you

❖ Some new (or old) discomforts may be (re)surfacing now, such as shortness of breath, heartburn, fatigue, varicose veins, and constipation (see pages 100 to 101).

your baby

❖ He measures approximately 17 inches (43 cm) from head to toe and weighs around 4 pounds (1.8 kg).

❖ His movements will change as he runs out of space in the womb. Expect more squirms and ripples than serious kicks.

❖ His digestive system is almost fully developed, although he still depends on the umbilical cord for nourishment.

"I want to give my daughter the leg up I never had. A savings account for whatever: her wedding, a down payment on her first home, extra funds to study abroad—something! I know most people pay for these on their own, but I want to be there for her when she's older, so that if she falls I know that I can catch her."

read all about it

While no two births are exactly the same, reading up on the stages of labor will give you a general road map of what to expect (see pages 114 to 115 and Parenting.com).

have a plan

Discuss with your doctor your preferences regarding the process of giving birth and interventions such as induction, pain relief, and episiotomy. (To read about birth plans, see page 122.)

Keep in mind, though, that circumstances may require something different. While you probably want to avoid unexpected procedures, like a c-section, it's always best to know what leads up to these interventions and what they entail, so that you're less likely to be caught off-guard if things don't go as planned.

true or false?

Braxton Hicks contractions are a mild tightening of the uterus that generally occur throughout pregnancy, though they may increase in frequency and duration as your time draws near. These "false labor" contractions are irregular and either painless or mildly uncomfortable (not like real labor pains!), but they can fool you into thinking labor's started. Here's how to tell the difference (but call your doctor if you're still not sure).

false labor	true labor
Contractions may feel similar to menstrual cramps.	Contractions may feel similar to menstrual cramps.
Contractions are irregular, don't increase in frequency, and will often subside if you lie down or take a walk.	Contractions occur at regular intervals, gradually get closer together, feel stronger, last longer, may intensify if you shift position, and don't go away if you rest or engage in mild physical activity.
Contractions tend to be felt in the front of the abdomen.	Contractions start in the back and come around to the front, sometimes moving from top to bottom.
Contractions are not closely preceded or accompanied by other labor symptoms.	Contractions are usually accompanied or closely preceded by other physical indications of labor. For a list of "labor clues," see page 118.

week 33

you

❖ You're gaining about a pound (.5 kg) a week.

❖ Because your growing baby is pressing up against your stomach, hampering digestion, gas and heartburn may accompany eating.

your baby

❖ She measures around 17½ inches (44 cm) from head to toe and weighs as much as 4½ pounds (2 kg).

❖ To practice breathing, your baby inhales amniotic fluid.

❖ Rapid eye movements suggest that your baby is dreaming.

mom to mom

"My hips and back have been aching so badly! I went to take my boys and the dog for a walk the other night, and we made it four blocks before I told them we had to turn around. My oldest son told me I could ride on his Power Wheels with him."

breastfeeding basics

Nursing your baby has many positives: it's a great way to bond with your baby; it's sterile, always ready, and free; and even a little bit of breastfeeding offers health benefits to you and your baby. Research shows that breastfed babies have fewer respiratory and ear infections and a lower risk of asthma and diabetes. Moms who breastfeed may lose postpartum pounds more quickly and enjoy a reduced risk of breast cancer and osteoporosis.

The American Academy of Pediatrics (AAP) recommends that babies receive breast milk exclusively for the first six months, and then in conjunction with solid foods up to a year, or longer if you desire. For personal, practical, or medical reasons, you may opt to supplement with formula or wean your baby before six months.

Keep in mind that breastfeeding often has a steep learning curve. Consider signing up for a breastfeeding class or reading a book on the subject now. If you need help, resources include lactation consultants, postpartum doulas, support groups, online forums, and other moms. (Also see pages 83 and 130.)

here's the formula

Not all new moms can or want to breastfeed. Careful government regulations ensure that domestic infant formulas are nutritious and safe. Your baby will do fine if you supplement with formula or feed him formula full-time. Here's what else you need to know:

❖ Formula comes in cow's milk, soy, hypoallergenic, and lactose-free formulations. Talk to your baby's pediatrician about the right type of formula for your baby.

❖ Varieties include ready-to-drink, liquid concentrate, or powder. Powder is the most economical choice but needs to be carefully prepared before feeding.

❖ Made to mimic breast milk, formula often contains healthy fats like DHA and ARA, which foster brain and nerve development.

vitamin D alert

The American Academy of Pediatrics recommends infants receive 400 IU of vitamin D daily. Babies drinking 32 ounces (1 l) of formula, which is enriched, a day will get enough vitamin D to meet this guideline. Babies drinking exclusively breast milk, however, won't. If you breastfeed, talk to your pediatrician about using vitamin D supplements.

got strep?

You'll soon be screened for the Group B streptococcus (GBS) virus. If passed to a baby during delivery, GBS can cause meningitis, pneumonia, or even death. If you test positive, don't panic. Up to 30 percent of pregnant women carry the virus. During delivery, you will receive antibiotics to protect your baby from contracting the virus.

week 34

you

❖ You may feel numbness or tingling in the pelvic area due to pressure from your growing baby.

❖ You're probably having mild contractions now, even if you can't feel them yet!

❖ If you take a non-stress test (see page 109), you'll see your contractions on a monitoring strip and hear the corresponding changes in your baby's heart rate.

your baby

❖ He measures approximately 18 inches (46 cm) from head to toe and may weigh as much as 5¼ pounds (2.4 kg).

❖ Your baby will open and close his eyes more now that your uterine and abdominal walls are stretching and getting thinner, allowing more light into the womb.

mom
to
mom

"I love breastfeeding! My breasts are good at what they do. It is an amazing and very difficult thing. But then again, so is childbirth. Painstakingly, I did it anyway, and I got through it."

will you have a c-section?

Some moms-to-be have scheduled cesarean sections because of known medical issues. For others, a c-section, if it happens, comes as an unexpected change in plans. About one-quarter to one-third of all U. S. hospital deliveries are c-sections, so even if you have had a healthy pregnancy and are making plans for a vaginal delivery, you could still end up having an unplanned cesarean. Just in case, it's important to familiarize yourself with the reasons for and details of the procedure.

Your doctor may want to schedule a c-section if your baby is breech or in a sideways position, if you're carrying multiples, or if you have a health issue such as preeclampsia (pregnancy-induced hypertension). An emergency surgical delivery may become necessary if your baby shows signs of distress during labor, such as heart-rate changes that indicate a problem with the umbilical cord or placenta. An excessively long labor that does not progress can also lead to surgical intervention.

To prepare yourself, attend a birth-preparation class or watch a birth video that covers c-sections, read up on the procedure, and talk to your doctor about the procedure.

recovery

If you end up having a c-section, expect a longer recovery. A c-section is major abdominal surgery—not only was your uterus cut, but so were the layers of muscle, fat, and skin above it. That's nothing to sneeze at (and sneezing, as well as coughing and laughing, can hurt, so be careful!).

If you're having a scheduled c-section, here are a few things you can plan for:

❖ You'll want to avoid stairs for a few weeks after delivery, if possible.

❖ You also won't be driving during that time, so try to make alternative arrangements in advance.

❖ Enlist help at home so you can focus on feeding your baby and healing your body.

don't make the cut

While episiotomies were once routine, research shows they frequently don't help and can actually make natural tearing (as well as recovery) worse. Ask your doctor how often he performs episiotomies, and discuss how you can work together to avoid one.

what's that wet?

Despite what you've seen on TV, water breaking prior to labor happens only about 10 percent of the time. When it does, there's not always a big gush—it may be more of a trickle. If your water breaks, call your doctor. You're at higher risk of infection, so if labor doesn't start naturally, you may need to be induced.

week 35

you

❖ Clear or yellowish fluid may be leaking from your nipples. That's *colostrum*, the early milk that your breasts produce in the first few days of your baby's life.

❖ You may be feeling even more fatigued now; give yourself permission to cut back and take breaks.

your baby

❖ She measures approximately 18½ inches (47 cm) from head to toe and weighs as much as 5½ pounds (2.5 kg).

❖ Nearly full term, her risk of complications, if she were born now, would be low.

❖ Her skull bones are soft and pliable to make her trip down the birth canal easier.

mom to mom

"I was always under the impression that you would 'know' when your water broke. They checked me at the hospital to see if it had broken, which involved putting a piece of litmus paper or something down there and made me cough. The fluid that touched the paper made it change colors, which meant it had broken—or, as the doctor said, 'leaked.'"

in the bag

Getting your hospital bag ready soon makes it easier to get out the door when it's time to go. Use the list on page 119 to guide you.

Ask the hospital about what's available in the labor and delivery rooms, for example, a birthing ball or a shower. Also, check to see if items like a cell phone, video camera, and laptop are allowed.

solo time

Take advantage of any free time. You'll appreciate the "me" time soon, since it turns into "we" time once your baby arrives. See the latest movies, read books or magazines you've been meaning to get to, or finish craft projects. Do whatever it is that *you* like to do.

the power of touch

Ah, massage. There's nothing like touch to soothe many pregnancy-related aches—including lower back pain and *sciatica* (lower back, butt, and leg pain caused by nerve compression). Ask your partner to practice these moves on you now—they can provide relief during labor, too. Or splurge on a professional prenatal massage.

❖ Gently rub your back, neck, arms, and legs using a rich massage oil or moisturizer—while you're lying on your left side.

❖ Press a tennis ball into your lower back while you are seated in a chair facing a bed, leaning forward over a stack of pillows.

❖ If you have a professional prenatal massage, a therapist will prop you up with pillows or use a table with a hole in the center to accommodate your belly. The pressure of her hands should be light, especially around the abdominal area.

❖ Be sure your partner or therapist avoids certain "trigger points" considered in acupressure to induce uterine contractions. These spots will feel extra-tender to the touch. They include the point between your thumb and index finger, your inner calf above the ankle, the top of your shoulder between the joint and your neck, and the back of your foot just above your heel.

wind down from work

Whether you plan to work right up until you feel the first contraction or begin your maternity leave sometime soon, bear in mind that you may not be able to plan it precisely.

For that reason, spend part of every day at work taking care of tasks left hanging, answering messages, organizing your work area, and leaving instructions for whoever is covering for you in your absence.

The more organized you are, the more relaxed you'll feel about leaving (especially if you have to go in a hurry!), and the more appreciative your boss will be.

week 36

you

❖ If you haven't already, you may be experiencing *sciatica* (lower back, butt, and leg pain caused by nerve compression). See page 50 for helpful massage techniques.

❖ As early as this week, you could lose your mucous plug—the thick protective barrier over your cervix.

❖ Your doctor will start seeing you weekly.

your baby

❖ He measures approximately 19 inches (48 cm) from head to toe and weighs about 6 pounds (2.7 kg).

❖ Your baby is putting on more fat, which will help keep him warm and regulate his body temperature once he's outside the womb.

mom to mom

"My doctor says I could have two to four weeks left to go. But, oh, the waddling! It started this week, and I feel like a beached whale as I move from place to place. Dear hubby thinks it's the funniest thing to watch me try to get up from the couch after watching TV. Glad he's amused!"

69

feathering the nest

In the coming weeks, you may find yourself overwhelmed by a sudden urge to get things done in preparation for your baby's arrival. Some moms-to-be sort and fold baby clothes; others get obsessed with nursery decorating details or even arranging the linen closet. A few things to remember about this common third-trimester phenomenon:

❖ Nesting is a natural response to impending motherhood.

❖ The physical act of nesting can help channel some of the nervous energy you may have about parenting responsibilities.

❖ Accomplishing tasks around your home may help you feel more in control.

❖ While you're rearranging for the umpteenth time, try to remember to take breaks. Also don't lift anything heavy.

❖ Keep your distance from paint or cleaning fumes and use nontoxic cleaning products. Hire help or pass tasks on to your partner, a family member, or a friend.

on the ball

A birthing or exercise ball—think big beach ball, only stronger—is a great tool for expecting moms. You can pick one up at a sporting goods store or online. Simply sitting on it can alter your posture, easing strain on your back and hips.

Try this: With the ball pushed up against a wall so it won't roll, turn your back to the ball, plant your feet wider than hip width apart, and sit down on the center of the top of the ball. Just sit, gently bounce in place, or slowly roll the ball under your hips from side to side.

As you get closer to your due date, bouncing on a birthing ball may help move your baby into position for birth. Many hospitals also offer birthing balls to moms during early labor so they can change position and reduce pain, particularly from back labor. If your hospital doesn't, you may want to bring your own (see page 119 for more about what to pack for the hospital).

week 37

you

❖ You may feel like your baby is about to drop out of you when you walk. (She won't!)

❖ At this week's checkup, your health practitioner will check to see if your cervix is effacing (thinning out) and dilating (opening up by tiny increments measured in centimeters) in preparation for labor (see page 114).

❖ Your weight may level off or even decrease by a pound or two—don't worry. The baby isn't losing weight.

your baby

❖ Your baby measures as much as 19½ inches (50 cm) from head to toe and weighs up to 7 pounds (3 kg).

❖ Considered full term this week, your baby may arrive any day.

mom to mom

"Much to our surprise, my dog thought that the baby was the most wonderful thing on Earth. The first week we had the baby home, my dog would run to the baby's room when he started crying, then run back to me with a look of 'Hurry up! He needs you!' on his little doggy face."

what a mess!

Birth is a beautiful thing, in theory. In reality, it's messy. Beforehand, your mucous plug (a gelatinous glob) will come out, all at once or in pieces, as will a mucous discharge tinged with blood, aka "bloody show." During active labor, you may throw up or poop as you push. It's because the rectum and birth canal are parallel. You'll be too busy to care, and, in any case, it's nothing labor nurses haven't seen and cleaned up briskly before!

helping nature along

Some babies need a little urging to emerge. Your doctor may use forceps (think giant salad tongs) or vacuum extraction (gentle suction) to help ease your baby out. You may want to talk to your doctor about the situations where these techniques can be useful.

labor with an epidural . . .

Epidural anesthesia is by far the most common medical pain-relief option. The procedure delivers medication through a catheter into a space near the spine, reducing or eliminating labor pain while allowing you to remain awake and alert.

The catheter allows the anesthesiologist to adjust the strength and frequency of the doses. On the downside, once you have that in, you're confined to lying in bed. Also, getting an epidural can lower your blood pressure and slow labor, increasing your chance of needing further interventions such as Pitocin, a synthetic hormone used to induce or speed labor. The numbness can make pushing more difficult. Potential side effects include headache, back soreness, itching, mild fever, and trembling.

A lower-dose or "walking" epidural may leave you with more sensation in your hips and legs, which can make pushing easier (the name is misleading—you won't get up and walk around). The anesthesiologist can also decrease the dose's strength to allow you to feel more sensation when it's time to push. Talk to your doctor about your options and preferences.

. . . and without

Even if you plan to have an epidural at the hospital, nonmedical "comfort" strategies may come in handy in early labor. Here are some suggestions (also see page 121), but see what you want in the moment. For instance, a massage may sound good to you now and may absolutely not be what you want during a contraction.

❖ Deep cleansing breaths, as well as more rapid ones

❖ Movement: walking, kneeling, rocking your pelvis

❖ Verbal encouragement from your partner, birth coach, nurse (see page 120)

❖ Massage on your hands, temples, back, feet (see page 68)

❖ Relaxing or energizing music

❖ A warm shower or bath

week 38

you

❖ You might be breathing easier now and have less heartburn since your baby's head has probably dropped down and shifted into the birth canal.

❖ For the same reason, the feeling of pressure on your groin, thighs, and bladder may increase.

your baby

❖ He measures approximately 20 inches (51 cm) from head to toe and weighs about 7½ pounds (3.4 kg).

❖ The lanugo (see page 27) and *vernix caseosa* (see page 37) have probably shed, leaving the soft skin you'll touch when he's born.

❖ His lungs and vocal chords are all ready for the first wail he'll make after delivery.

mom to mom

"My epidural was actually a little weak when I had my third baby, but I really enjoyed being able to 'experience' birth more. For my first two deliveries, I didn't feel anything. This time, I could feel some pressure during the contractions, and I was able to feel him being born. Uncomfortable, not painful, and totally exhilarating!"

extra-credit prep

Other things you may want to do that could make the first months of motherhood run more smoothly include:

❖ Arrange for bills to be paid automatically.

❖ Sign up for a grocery delivery service.

❖ Collect local takeout and delivery menus.

❖ Stock up on different size batteries for the bouncy seat, swing, mobile, etc.

speed dial

Gather the numbers of people—your pediatrician and a lactation consultant, for instance—who could be a resource for you during those challenging early weeks. Enter these in your phone now, so you'll be ready once you bring your baby home.

are you ready?

It's easy to put off certain to-dos. But since your baby could come anytime now, it's good to make sure all systems are a go as soon as possible. Here's a checklist of pre-baby steps to take:

○ Install your infant car safety seat (see page 85).

○ Check smoke detectors and carbon monoxide detectors.

○ Pack your hospital bag (see page 119).

○ Plan how to contact your partner when you go into labor.

○ Stock up on diaper supplies (see page 82).

○ Wash, dry, and sort some, but not all, of your newborn clothes (your baby may be smaller or bigger, so you may want to exchange some items).

○ If you're planning to breastfeed, buy nursing bras—two for now, because you will get bigger (see page 83).

○ Cook ahead and freeze some meals.

○ Buy household supplies (paper goods, detergent) in bulk.

○ Research and select a birth announcement (see page 124).

helping hands

While you're busy handling pre-baby tasks on your own, don't forget that there's a lot other people can do for you, now and—most important—after the birth. If friends or family offer help, sign 'em up! They can make and freeze meals, wash baby clothes, and shop for essentials. Later, these willing hands can help with household chores. If you can hire help, you have options; consider a house cleaner, a baby nurse, or a postpartum doula.

week 39

you

❖ Many moms-to-be feel pretty clumsy in the final weeks, so step carefully as you navigate stores, sidewalks, and stairs.

❖ You're probably thirstier lately, so be sure to drink plenty of fluids.

your baby

❖ Her length is probably about the same as last week, around 18 to 21½ inches (46 to 55 cm) from head to toe. Her weight may also be holding steady at about 6 to 9 pounds (2.7 to 4 kg).

❖ Her brain, one of the last organs to fully develop, is busy firing neurons.

"I read lists with loads of things you should take to the hospital with you. I packed everything they said and needed very few of them. For the baby, you need a going-home outfit and a car seat. Take a baby book so you can get the nurses to stamp the feet in when they're doing the birth certificate."

nature's labor starters

Family and friends—even strangers—will probably suggest these natural labor-inducing strategies. Most have little or no scientific evidence to support their efficacy, but they can't hurt:

❖ Take a walk. Some women swear that a brisk stroll around the block got their contractions started.

❖ Jump in bed. Sex is a favorite labor inducer. There may be some truth to this one—prostaglandins, found in semen, could soften the cervix; arousal and orgasm also trigger the release of oxytocin, the same brain chemical released during labor.

❖ Try nipple stimulation. This action also releases oxytocin, which could bring on contractions. Check with your doctor first: Some feel this technique is safest if you're already being monitored at a hospital, since it can bring on contractions quickly.

time for induction

Sometimes labor needs a little help getting started. The most common way for your doctor to give things a push medically is administering intravenous Pitocin (a synthetic form of the contraction-triggering hormone oxytocin). Your doctor can also rupture the membranes that bind your amniotic sac to the uterine wall, prescribe synthetic prostaglandin gels, or break your water.

Issues that can lead your doctor to consider inducing labor include high blood pressure, low amniotic fluid volume, high fetal weight, or evidence of fetal distress. Induction may also be considered if your water breaks but contractions don't start on their own, or your pregnancy continues past forty-two weeks.

Some women would like to be induced, even if no medical indicators are present. But the procedure is not one to be taken lightly. Pitocin brings on sudden, intense contractions, so pain medication is a must for many women. And since these powerful contractions can cause fetal distress or even uterine rupture, constant electronic fetal monitoring is needed. There is also the potential for longer labor, which is more likely to result in medical interventions, such as a c-section. Go over the pros and cons carefully with your doctor before making this decision.

baby bonding

You probably expect to fall in love with your baby at first sight, and many new moms do. But if you don't immediately, that's normal, too. After giving birth, huge hormonal changes, a tough pregnancy or labor, or worries about taking care of your baby can influence your emotions in ways you may not expect.

Don't worry—bonding will happen, and neither you nor your baby will suffer any consequences if you don't have a thunderbolt moment. If you continue to feel anxious, fearful, or sad (all normal emotions), talk to your doctor.

week 40+

you

❖ While you've reached your due date, you won't technically be overdue for another two weeks.

❖ Back pain, nausea, or diarrhea may reappear or increase now as your body prepares for labor.

your baby

❖ Average length and weight are 20 inches (51 cm) from head to toe and 7½ pounds (3.4 kg). But results may differ by 4 inches (10.2 cm) and 3 pounds (1.4 kg) on either side!

❖ At birth, he may have a cone-shaped head, puffy eyes, and a coating of amniotic fluid and blood.

❖ His vision will be blurry, but he'll recognize the sound of your voice right away.

mom to mom

"When having contractions, try to get up and walk around. I know it's hard to do, but that helped me get things moving a little faster with my son. With every contraction, I walked, even if it hurt really bad. Gravity is our friend during labor!"

gear

gear

How can one tiny person require so much stuff? Well, they don't—or not all of it, anyway. This section will help you figure out what you really need and when you need it. For now, you can zero in on the absolute essentials—the stuff that will get you through those first few months with your newborn (also see page 40). And you don't have to go it alone. Veteran parents can often help out with their recommendations. Delegate to your partner, too. Gear-heads get into test-driving bigger equipment such as car seats and strollers.

Here, we break down the categories—from nursery to feeding to traveling, and everything in between. You'll also find advice on what to buy new and what's fine to score secondhand or borrow. Finally, a master checklist will keep it all organized. Happy shopping!

What do you already have?

_____

_____

_____

_____

What are you most excited about getting?

_____

_____

_____

_____

_____

crib notes

It's best to buy a new crib: It will meet current safety standards (slats no more than 2⅜ inches [6 cm] apart, for instance), and you'll get all the pieces and instructions, as well as a warranty. *Note:* It's good to order furniture in your second trimester—it can take months to arrive. New cribs range from $100 to over $1,000. You pay extra for fancier styles, but look for these key fixtures:

❖ Sturdy structure: Give the crib a good shake both in the store and after you put it together at home to check that screws, brackets, and joints are stable and quiet.

❖ Firm, new mattress: Most crib mattresses are sold separately. Even if you're using a hand-me-down crib, get a new mattress; researchers have established a link between used mattresses and sudden infant death syndrome (SIDS). The mattress should fit snugly in the crib. If you can fit more than two fingers between the mattress and crib frame, it's not snug enough.

❖ Safe design: Avoid cribs with corner posts (clothing can get caught) or decorative cutouts (your baby can get a limb stuck).

❖ Stationary sides: Drop-down sides make getting your baby in and out easier, but recalls have raised concerns about their safety. For now, most experts recommend buying a crib with stationary sides until more stringent standards are established.

❖ Height-adjustable mattress: The highest level makes picking up a newborn easier. You lower it in stages as your baby starts pushing herself up.

❖ Toddler-bed conversion: Some cribs can convert, but the kits, often sold separately, can be expensive. This feature might not be as important if you're planning to have another baby in the next couple of years and will need a crib again.

Think twice about a used crib—your baby will spend more time there than anyplace else, and you want it to be as safe as possible. Never use a crib made before the 1990s, when the current safety standards were established. While the newer the better, if you use a gently used hand-me-down crib, consult the Consumer Product Safety Commission's website, CPSC.gov, for product recalls.

don't bump

Bumper pads and their fasteners may pose a suffocation or strangulation hazard. If you choose to use a bumper pad, select one that's firm and cut off any excess ties after you've secured it, or opt for a breathable mesh bumper. Remove it when your baby can push up on his hands and knees, about 5 months.

become a fan

Running a fan in your baby's room may reduce the risk of sudden infant death syndrome (SIDS)—and the "white noise" it creates may also help your baby sleep! Also don't overheat the nursery: The recommended range is 68° to 72° F (20° to 22.2° C).

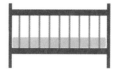

sleep smarts

Some nursing moms find that having their newborns sleep in the same room with them makes night feedings easier. However, the American Academy of Pediatrics (AAP) does not recommend co-sleeping (having your child sleep in your bed with you), due to safety issues including an increased risk of sudden infant death syndrome (SIDS). Better: having your baby close by but not in an adult bed. Your options:

❖ Move the crib into your bedroom. If space is an issue, opt for a traditional bassinet or cradle (though your baby will outgrow these cozy sleepers at about 15 pounds or so, depending on the design).

❖ Consider a three-sided bassinet that attaches to the side of your bed, known as a "co-sleeper."

❖ Pick up a play yard. Some of these foldable structures come with a bassinet attachment that's just right for a newborn. Later on, you can use it as a travel crib or playpen (see page 87).

❖ Settle her in her own digs. It's fine for your newborn to sleep in her crib in her nursery. Trust us; you'll hear her!

❖ Wing it. Many newborns nap soundly in a bouncy seat, car seat, or baby swing, so don't stress about the "right" place, especially in the early months before her sleep patterns are organized. Just be sure that someone always stays with her whenever she's in a bouncy seat, car seat, or swing, whether she's asleep or awake.

keep it clear

Wherever your baby sleeps, keep loose blankets and soft toys out. They pose a suffocation and sudden infant death syndrome (SIDS) risk. Use a sleep sack to keep her warm.

wrap me up

Many infants love being swaddled: cozily wrapped up in a blanket. Some even sleep better that way. Best types for the job are thin, light, and larger than receiving blankets. You can also buy specially designed swaddling blankets. Ask a hospital nurse to show you how it's done before you go home—or check out our how-to video on Parenting.com.

"She hated her bassinet, so we set up her crib in our room. We let her sleep like that for about two months, and then moved the crib back into her room. I let her play in her room from the day we brought her home, though, so she was used to the room itself. It probably sounds silly since she was just a little newborn, but I was afraid she would wake up and wonder, 'Where am I? Whaaa!'"

bum wrapping

Cloth? Disposable? A bit of both? Your diaper options are many. If you choose to go the cloth route, you can wash them at home yourself or use a pick-up-and-drop-off diaper service. You can buy all-in-ones that combine diaper and cover, or pre-folded cloth diapers you use with separate covers. Or you could head to the store for one of dozens of disposable variations, including some that are kinder to the environment. Bottom line: Choose what works best for your lifestyle.

Whatever the method, have enough diapers on hand for the first week—you'll want to have at least eighty ready at home, if you're using disposables. Don't buy too many diapers in a newborn size, though; babies rapidly grow out of them. Brands fit differently, so it may take a diaper blowout or two before you can figure out which one is right for your baby! Less-expensive warehouse or store brands can definitely be as good as name brands, but not always, so experiment.

All you really need to change a diaper is a mat and a safe spot; you don't have to purchase a changing table. But it is convenient to have an area designated for diaper duty so all your supplies are in one place. If you decide to buy a ready-made table, look for one that can do duty as a storage unit or dresser.

pacify me

Pacifiers fell out of favor for a while, but new research linking their use to a reduced risk of sudden infant death syndrome (SIDS) has put them front and center again. If you offer a pacifier to your baby, keep in mind:

❖ While some lactation experts believe pacifiers interfere with establishing breastfeeding, research doesn't support that claim.

❖ Not all babies love 'em. Offer it, but you can't always force it.

❖ Test out different shapes, sizes, and materials to determine what works for your baby. Natural rubber is an allergen-free, chemical-free option.

the poop on goop

Diaper rash is always an occupational hazard. To prevent and treat it, use a diaper cream to create a moisture barrier (this reduces the friction that helps trigger rash). Avoid baby powder—studies show it may be harmful to baby's lungs. (See page 91 for a complete list of diaper supplies.)

laundry quandary

Laundry detergent made just for baby things isn't necessary. Just be sure whatever detergent you choose is hypoallergenic, contains no chlorine or phosphates, and is free of dyes or fragrances. Plan to soak stained items (poop, spit-up, breast milk, etc.) right away with detergent or a stain remover.

breastfeeding

All you need are your breasts, right? Not exactly. Supporting equipment starts with a well-fitting cotton nursing bra. The pressure from a too-tight bra can lead to a blocked duct or a breast infection. Get fitted and purchase two a few weeks before you're due. Then get re-fitted and stock up a couple of weeks after birth when breast swelling subsides. Stretchy, cotton nursing bras or tanks also offer a comfortable round-the-clock option.

Nursing pads absorb leakage, but change them often to help avoid yeast infections. Also, have pure-lanolin ointment on hand to prevent and treat cracked nipples. (For more tips, see page 130.)

Using a breast pump allows you to express milk to store for later or to share feeding duties. A pump is a must-have if you go back to work and continue to nurse. Pumping briefly before nursing can help your baby latch on and relieve engorgement—but be careful, too much pumping can have the opposite effect. Some mothers pump exclusively if their babies have trouble nursing. Electric pumps are easier to use than manual ones. Usually used on the advice of a doctor or lactation consultant, hospital-grade pumps are the most efficient—and expensive—but you can rent one.

rock the bottle

Whether breast milk or formula goes in it, the advice is the same:

❖ Newborns consume only a few ounces at a time, so start with small bottles (4 to 5 ounces or .1 to .15 l) and low-flow nipples. You might have to try different designs and brands to find one with a shape and flow rate that your infant will accept.

❖ Clear, hard plastic bottles are fast becoming a no-no because of concerns about exposing infants to the chemical Bisphenol A (BPA), which these bottles often contain. To err on the side of caution, use BPA-free plastic bottles or bottle systems with soft, disposable plastic liners.

❖ Get a bottle brush and drying rack, but skip a fancy sterilizer; a dishwasher with a basket for nipples and rings is fine. You'll also need a cold pack and insulated bag for toting formula on the go.

clean up

You can bathe your newborn in an infant tub or in the sink. Have on hand: all-in-one baby wash, shampoo, cotton balls, washcloths, a hooded towel, and baby lotion for after a bath.

medicine cabinet

Stock these essential health-care items before you bring your baby home (for a more detailed list, see page 91):

❖ Digital rectal thermometer and covers or alcohol wipes

❖ Nasal aspirator (nose-suction bulb), which the hospital may provide

❖ Infant acetaminophen (always read the label to make sure you get the infant—not kids—version!); never give aspirin, which can cause the rare and serious Reye's syndrome

baby on board

Get cracking now on buying and installing an infant car seat—you won't be able to take your baby home without it! Car seats with five-point harness systems are the safest. For your newborn, you need a rear-facing infant seat: She'll be in it until she's at least a year old and she weighs at least 20 pounds (9 kg). Most models can hold up to 22 to 30 pounds (10 to 13.6 kg), or you can buy a convertible car seat, which may go up to 35 pounds (16 kg) rear-facing and 40 to 65 pounds (18 to 29.5 kg) forward-facing.

It's best to buy a brand-new car seat to make sure that it meets the latest standards and you receive any recall notices. If you do borrow or buy one used, make sure that it has not been in a collision, confirm that it has not been recalled (find reports at CPSC.gov), and check that it fits in your car.

style options

Here are your basic car seat options. Whatever kind you opt for, always check the seat's weight and height limits, and get one with a removable, washable cover.

❖ A convertible car seat: The high weight and height limits mean your baby can use it until she's ready to graduate to a booster. The downside: They're big, and you can't carry them around.

❖ An infant seat: The biggest benefit is that it snaps into and out of a base installed in your car, so you can release the seat and carry a sleeping baby without disturbing her. An infant seat can also snap into a matching stroller or stroller frame. To share one seat between two cars, simply buy an extra base. The downside: Your baby will grow out of the seat eventually, and you'll need to move up to a bigger convertible model.

❖ An infant-seat-and-stroller combo: Called a travel system, this is a popular all-in-one option. Be sure you like the stroller the seat snaps into; after your baby outgrows the seat, he'll be using that stroller for a long time (see page 86).

safe at home

You'll want to begin childproofing at about six months—before your baby is crawling around. But for now, locking gates, gadgets, and gizmos are not necessary. What you should check: that you have functioning smoke and carbon monoxide detectors on each floor of your home, and that you have a fire extinguisher and know how to use it!

boiling point

Make sure you turn your home's water heater down to 120° F (49° C) to avoid accidental scalding.

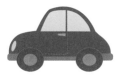

installation tips

The National Highway Traffic Safety Administration reports that a whopping 80 percent of children are improperly restrained in safety seats. Local police departments often offer free inspections. Visit NHTSA.gov to find a certified inspector near you.

❖ Install a car seat at a 45-degree angle. If it lies too flat, your baby could slide out between the straps; if it's too upright, her head could flop forward. If your model doesn't have an angle-adjuster, you can wedge a rolled towel to fit under the base.

❖ The carrying handle should be in the down position (behind your baby's head) for most infant seats when installed in a car. Check the manual.

❖ Put the harness straps in a rear-facing seat in slots at or *below* your baby's shoulders (note: they should be at or *above* shoulder level in a forward-facing seat) and the top of the harness clip at armpit level. The harness should lie snug and flat.

❖ The seat must be installed in the backseat—ideally in the middle—and tightly secured with a safety belt or with LATCH.

❖ If your model has a separate base, be sure the seat is snapped in firmly every time.

❖ When properly installed, all car seats will move less than an inch when you tug on them in any direction.

latch on

Lower Anchors and Tethers for Children (LATCH) is a system of metal rings and hooks that you can use instead of a safety belt to secure a car seat into a car. All models of car seats except boosters are required to have this hardware, and all vehicles manufactured after September 1, 2002 will have the corresponding hooks.

If you have an older car without the LATCH system however, don't worry. Properly anchoring a car seat with a safety belt as shown in a manufacturer's instructions is as safe as using LATCH. Having a car retrofitted is sometimes also an option.

rolling sideshow

Keeping your baby entertained in the car can be a challenge. Stow a plush ball, a cloth book, or other soft toy in the backseat. Some toys are designed to strap onto a car seat handle, which keeps them from getting dropped on the floor in transit. Busy boards attach to the back of the seat in front of him, with buttons and gizmos he can activate by kicking his feet. A mirror does double duty, giving him someone to look at, and giving you a view of your baby's reflection in your rearview mirror. Caution: Be extra vigilant when driving. A baby on board—especially a crying one—ups your distraction level.

strolling along

Shop for a stroller as carefully as you'd shop for a car. Seriously! There are so many types, and it's smart to get one that suits your lifestyle and needs. Some maneuver easily on urban streets; others are easy to fold and toss in the back of a minivan. You may even want more than one! The good news: You can easily find and buy gently used models from other stroller-happy parents.

Paramount for a newborn is a stroller that will support her fully reclined. Also consider things like the design and height of handles, canopy for sun-protection (and a peek-through window, so you can still see her), and onboard storage room.

❖ Many parents start with an infant car seat and a stroller frame that the seat snaps onto. Generally inexpensive, lightweight frames are easy to fold and toss in the trunk—a plus when you're recovering postpartum, especially after a c-section.

❖ A carriage-style stroller offers a bassinet that snaps into the frame or a regular seat that reclines fully.

❖ A travel system combines an infant car seat, a base that stays in the car, and a full-size stroller that the seat clicks into. Be sure to test-drive the stroller alone to see if you like it. These strollers can be heavy and cumbersome. Also note the car seat's weight limit (see page 84).

Once your baby can sit up, you'll have additional options:

❖ An umbrella stroller: So named for its small folded size, these are great for travel and maneuvering in tight spaces.

❖ A stand-alone full-size stroller: These are more cumbersome to transport but are perfect for frequent around-the-neighborhood walks. They often offer bells and whistles such as snack trays, roomy baskets, and cushy padding.

❖ An all-terrain stroller: Air-inflated wheels and shock-absorbers make these a smooth ride over rough surfaces, and they're light enough to make jogging or power-walking with your baby (check the manual for age or size limitations) feasible.

carry me

You'll spend a lot of time holding your baby close and walking him (and, no, it's not possible to spoil a newborn with too many cuddles!). Baby carriers can make this together time easier on your arms and back.

Fabric slings and wraps hold your baby snugly against your body. Other, more structured, carriers may fit in front, on your back, or both.

Look for adjustable straps, shoulder padding, a range of carrying configurations, and lumbar support. And make sure the material can be washed!

Try to borrow a few before buying to see which type feels most comfortable.

it's in the bag

Good news: You don't have to carry a cutesy diaper bag with rabbits and duckies unless you want to! These days, diaper bags are fashion items, and many are also gender neutral. Look for one that's durable, lightweight, washable, and has pockets for diapers, wipes, feeding supplies (insulated compartments are handy), and so on. Some hook onto strollers. A backpack style is also a good hands-free option. You may want a smaller one for quick errands and a more serious size for longer ventures.

savvy packing

Use this diaper-bag checklist to organize your new #1 accessory. In fact, you might want to copy it, or make your own custom list, and stash it in the bag to double-check before you go out. To help keep the bag packed and ready to go, replenish supplies every time you come home. You don't want to run out the door and find yourself at the mall with a messy diaper and no wipes!

- ○ Diapers
- ○ Wipes
- ○ Diaper cream
- ○ Changing pad
- ○ Hand sanitizer
- ○ Nursing pads, or bottle and formula
- ○ Burp cloth
- ○ Spare outfit (or two)
- ○ Toy and book
- ○ Pacifier and cover or carry-case (if using)
- ○ Plastic/waterproof bags (for dirty diapers or soiled clothes)
- ○ Baby-formula sunblock
- ○ Hat
- ○ Blankets (an extra makes a handy, clean play surface)

crib on-the-go

Whenever you travel, you can ensure that your baby has a safe place to sleep by bringing a play yard with a bassinet attachment or a portable crib.

There are also some smaller products made just for travel, such as the PeaPod, a mini pup tent that folds down to the size of a large dinner plate, with an inflatable mattress.

make it routine

It may sound ho-hum to you, but all babies love repetition. Establishing a predictable routine early on helps your baby fall asleep reliably. For example, read the same book and sing the same lullaby every evening at bedtime, to send a clear "nighty-night!" signal. To save your sanity, look for ones that you won't mind reading or singing many thousands of times over!

fluffy festival

Your baby will no doubt acquire a veritable zoo of plush toy animals. At first, he probably won't show any interest in them, and it's a mystery which ones he will bond with when he does get curious around 8 to 12 months. *Safety note:* Do not put stuffed animals or other soft toys in the crib (see page 81).

easy reader

Books with bright colors, high contrast, textures, and sounds will appeal to even newborn babies. Shiny surfaces, varied textures, and elements that crinkle or squeak are good, as well as flaps that lift to reveal surprises.

Babies generally like stories with rhythm, rhyme, repetition, and minimal words per page. Photos or illustrations of items found in your infant's world—babies, pets, balls—will also appeal. Board or cloth books will be easiest for your baby, in time, to hold and handle (and chew).

Here are a few good bedtime stories beyond Margaret Wise Brown's *Goodnight Moon* to start your library:

❖ *Say Goodnight* by Helen Oxenbury

❖ *I Love You As Much* by Laura Krauss Melmed

❖ *Time for Bed* by Mem Fox

❖ *The Little Quiet Book* by Katherine Ross

that funky music

At first, simple rhythmic sounds constitute music for your newborn—like your heartbeat or any kind of white noise (the hum of a fan, vacuum cleaner, or radio static). Studies have shown that songs you listened to while your baby was in utero may also be soothing now. Don't think it all has to be "baby" lullabies, though; folk, jazz, classical, even your favorite rock or pop tunes, can be surprising baby soothers. Experiment with your own music library. Who knows what'll become your baby's ideal song?

favorite playthings

Of course you want to teach and entertain your child. But to start, all she needs is the sound of your voice, the look on your face, and the sights, sounds, and smells of her home and the outside world. To her, everything is new! As she grows, you can add toys to stimulate her mind and occupy her hands—and feet, and mouth!

Small infants who can't yet manipulate toys will get the most out of objects with visual appeal or simple sound effects, such as the clacking of a rattle. Like with books, look for toys with contrasting colors, patterns, and textures: soft blocks, mobiles, and mirrors. Bath toys are optional: One rubber ducky will do for now.

If you get a mechanical mobile, make sure it's battery-operated. Otherwise, you'll be running into the nursery every three minutes to wind it. Also, remember to remove the mobile when your baby is able to push up on her hands and knees (at about 5 months) because it then becomes a strangulation risk.

choking hazards

One of your baby's major jobs will be to put everything in his mouth. That makes policing his playthings for choking hazards one of your major jobs. Any toy, part of a toy, or household object (such as coins) within your baby's reach that can fit inside a 1¾-inch (4.4 cm) diameter tube—about the size of a standard toilet paper roll—can get caught in his throat and cause him to choke. Also keep away from your baby:

❖ Items with buttons or magnets that can come loose

❖ Spherical objects approximately the size of a golf ball— 1¾ inches (4.4 cm) in diameter—or smaller

❖ Latex balloons, especially deflated ones

❖ Any crib toy with a string longer than 6 inches (15 cm), or any pull toy with a string longer than 12 inches (30.5 cm)

bouncing along

A bouncy seat with a toy bar can be entertaining for young babies who can't yet sit up unassisted. One with a vibrating function can help calm a fussy baby and lull him into the land of nod. The seats also offer a safe place to put your baby for a few minutes while you take a shower. Just keep him in the bathroom where you can see him.

let's swing

A swing can do double duty as an entertaining place for your baby and as a calming or sleep aid. The motion can be fun, and it imitates the comforting movement of the womb, which may rock your baby to sleep. Not all babies take to them, so try to borrow one to try out first. Never leave a baby unattended in a swing.

complete gear guide

NURSERY NEEDS

O crib (see page 80)

   o firm mattress

   o sheet protector or mattress pad

   o 3 fitted sheets (look for elastic all the way around, not just at the corners)

O dresser

O changing table (optional)

O changing pad with waist strap

O 3 changing pad covers

O fan (see page 80)

O rocking chair or glider

O monitor (unless you live in a small home)

optional gear

O bassinet or cradle (see page 81)

   o 3 size-specific fitted sheets

O Portable crib or play yard with bassinet attachment (see page 87)

   o 3 size-specific fitted sheets

O musical mobile

O glow-in-the-dark clock

O pacifiers (see page 82)

ENTERTAINMENT

O books (see page 88)

O toys (see page 89)

O bouncy seat (see page 89)

O swing (see page 89)

ON-THE-GO GEAR

O car seat (see page 84)

O stroller that allows your newborn to fully recline (see page 86)

optional gear

O snap-in carrier frame for infant car seat

O sling or front carrier (see page 86)

LAYETTE

O homecoming outfit

O 6 to 8 snap-bottom undershirts

O 4 coveralls (one-piece footed outfits)

O 3 to 5 side-snap undershirts

O 3 shirt-and-pant sets

O sweater or sweatshirt

O 6 pairs of socks

O 8 sleep gowns with elastic bottoms or coverall pajamas

O 4 sleep sacks or blanket sleepers

O 4 receiving blankets

O 2 swaddling blankets (see page 81)

O lots of burp cloths and bibs

depending on the weather

O jacket, coat, or snowsuit

O knit hat

O brimmed sun hat

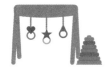

DIAPERS

O cloth or disposable diapers (see page 82)

O wipes (unscented for newborns)

O diaper pail or disposal unit and liners

O diaper cream (see page 82)

O diaper bag (see page 87 for a packing list) and portable changing pad

BATHING AND GROOMING

O infant tub (optional)

O all-in-one baby wash/shampoo

O baby lotion

O cotton balls

O 4 baby washcloths

O 2 large infant towels with hoods

O baby nail scissors or clippers

MEDICINE CABINET

O digital rectal thermometer

o covers or alcohol wipes for cleaning

O nasal aspirator

O saline spray or drops

O vaporizer

O infant acetaminophen (see page 83)

O baby sunblock

SAFETY

O smoke detectors

O fire extinguisher

O carbon monoxide detector

BREASTFEEDING

O 2 fitted nursing bras (see page 83)

O several stretchy nursing bras or tanks

O disposable or washable nursing pads

O pure-lanolin ointment

O nursing pillow

O breast pump (see page 83)

O 2 bottles and nipples

O freezer storage bags

O formula for emergencies

BOTTLE-FEEDING

O formula (see page 64)

O 6 to 8 small bottles and nipples (see page 83)

O disposable bottle liners (if planning to use)

O bottle brush (with nipple brush)

O bottle-drying rack

O dishwasher basket for nipples and rings

O insulated bottle bag and cold pack

shopping notes

sign up

Don't feel it's somehow pushy to register for baby things you want and need. If you're having a baby shower, guests will be relieved to have the guesswork taken out of gift giving. Tips: Register at more than one place and be sure there are both store and online options for gift buyers. Select items at all price points. And express your thanks with a brief, heartfelt, handwritten note as soon as you can! Keep track of gifts, givers, and thank-yous with the gift list on pages 94 to 95.

Use these pages to keep track of your buying options—such as stroller makes and models, crib prices, and favorite stores and websites. Paste in paint swatches for the nursery walls or scraps of fabric for curtains. Or just jot down baby names!

_____

_____

_____

_____

_____

_____

_____

_____

_____

_____

gifts and thank-yous

gift	from	thank-you sent ✓

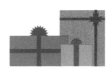

gift	from	thank-you sent ✓

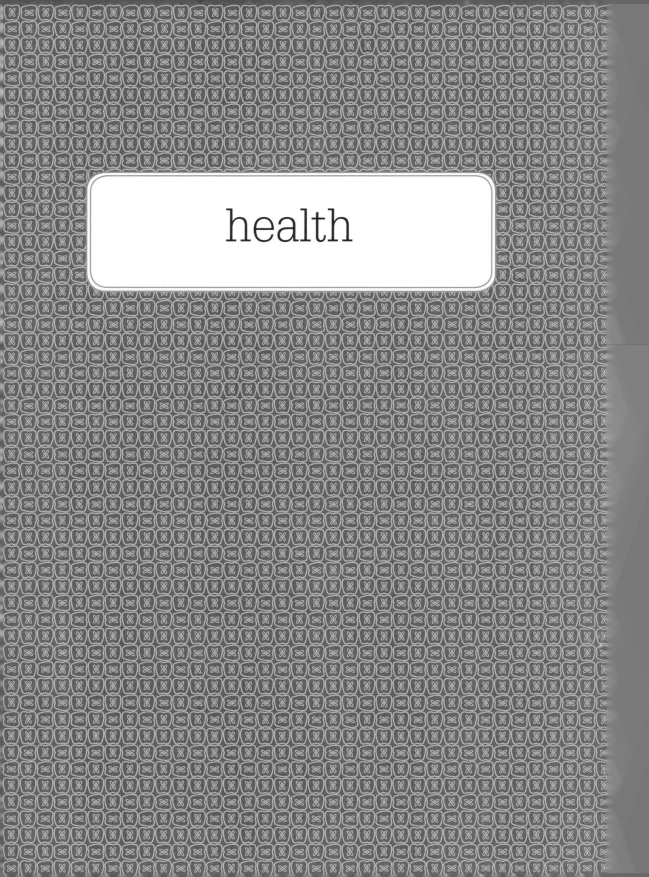

health

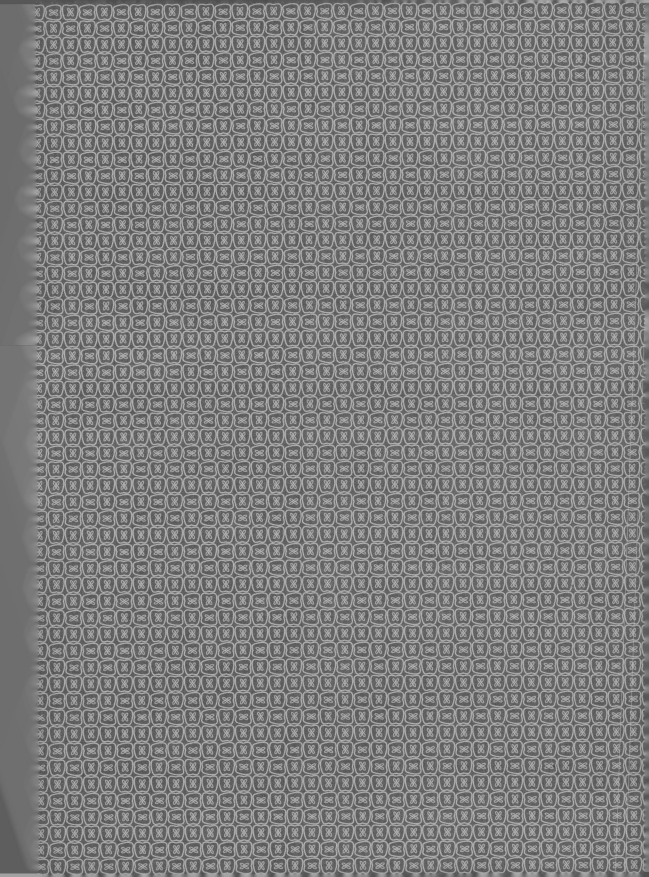

health

Do you find yourself being super health conscious now? It's no wonder; there's nothing like that bump expanding in front of you to remind you that everything you do, you now do for two. This section is all about health: helping demystify common concerns, like what to eat and what to avoid; giving you a run-down on the usual battery of prenatal tests; and explaining the multitude of pregnancy symptoms, including many that can be downright embarrassing, uncomfortable, or just plain gross. Check out our "Ick! What's that?" lists on pages 100 to 101 and 134 to 135 to find out what's going on and how to deal with it. You'll also find questions to ask prospective health-care providers for you and your baby.

Pregnancy is an important time to focus on your health—for your sake as well as for your baby's. Who knows: Some good pregnancy habits may last into your life as a new mom!

Which changes in your body have been the biggest surprise so far?

_____

_____

_____

_____

What are some of the best and worst parts about your pregnant body?

_____

_____

_____

_____

food-safety cheat sheet

RAW OR UNDERCOOKED FOOD
Some raw foods can cause listeriosis, salmonellosis, and other illnesses that,
though very rare, can lead to miscarriage or serious health problems for your baby.

what's okay
- ✓ thoroughly cooked meats, poultry, and seafood (also see below)
- ✓ vegetarian sushi
- ✓ deli meats (cold cuts) and hotdogs that have been heated to steaming
- ✓ canned or shelf-stable patés and meat spreads

what to avoid
- ✘ raw or undercooked meats, poultry, and seafood
- ✘ raw sprouts, including radish
- ✘ raw or undercooked eggs (such as in some salad dressings and protein shakes)

FISH
Certain fish contain high levels of mercury, which can contribute to developmental
delays. Farm-raised fish may be contaminated with polychlorinated biphenyls
(PCBs), which are cancer-causing agents, and other toxins.

what's okay
- ✓ canned or shelf-stable salmon
- ✓ up to 12 ounces (340 g) a week of:
  - catfish
  - cod
  - flounder
  - haddock
  - ocean perch
  - pollack
  - wild salmon (not farm-raised)
  - sardines
  - sea bass
  - shrimp
  - snapper
  - sole
  - tilapia
  - canned "light" tuna (up to 6 ounces or 170 g)

what to avoid
- ✘ king mackerel
- ✘ shark
- ✘ raw shellfish
- ✘ smoked seafood (refrigerated lox, trout, whitefish) unless cooked in another dish
- ✘ raw sushi
- ✘ swordfish
- ✘ tilefish
- ✘ canned albacore tuna
- ✘ fresh tuna

CHEESE AND DAIRY PRODUCTS

Raw or unpasteurized dairy products can cause illnesses such as listeriosis and salmonellosis.

what's okay
- ✓ pasteurized milk, yogurts, and soft cheeses
- ✓ well-cooked (that is, not runny) eggs
- ✓ hard cheeses

what to avoid
- ✗ raw milk and any dairy products (cheese, yogurt) made with raw milk
- ✗ unpasteurized soft cheeses, such as Brie, feta, Chèvre, Camembert, blue cheese, Roquefort, and Mexican-style queso blanco or fresco
- ✗ uncooked foods made with raw egg, such as some salad dressings and protein shakes

CAFFEINE/HERBAL TEAS

Research has linked caffeine to a higher rate of miscarriage; it can cross the placenta and affect fetal heart rate and respiration. Some herbs may cause adverse reactions.

what's okay
- ✓ less than 200 milligrams of caffeine a day (an 8-ounce cup of coffee has about 150 mg, a 12-ounce soda about 50 mg, and an 8-ounce cup of black tea about 40 mg; see page 8)
- ✓ flavored decaf teas in filter bags (citrus, ginger, or peppermint)

what to avoid
- ✗ teas made with goldenseal, black or blue cohosh, ephedra, dong quai, feverfew, juniper, pennyroyal, St. John's wort, rosemary, or thuja
- ✗ green tea during the first trimester, then in moderation

ARTIFICIAL SWEETENERS

There's no proof that artificial sweeteners cause harm to babies in utero; however, some experts caution against them.

what's okay
- ✓ aspartame and sucralose in moderate amounts

what to avoid
- ✗ saccharin (check with your doctor)
- ✗ drinking lots of diet drinks instead of healthier fluids such as water, milk, or juice

"ick! what's that?"

marked up

In addition to stretch marks, all manner of streaks and splotches may show up on your skin. There might be the linea nigra drawing itself down your belly (see page 21), the "mask of pregnancy" spreading across your face (see page 12), and spider veins crawling up your arms, chest, neck, or face. The usual suspects—hormones and extra blood flow—are to blame. Don't worry: The dark patches and veins usually fade postpartum.

Q. What's that thick discharge?

A. Sticky white or pale yellow discharge, called *leukorrhea*, can be constant during pregnancy. You can wear a lightweight sanitary pad. Do not douche. Talk to your doctor if the discharge develops a foul odor, itches, burns, or becomes greenish yellow or very thick or watery; those symptoms can be signs of an infection.

Q. Why am I farting so much?

A. Thanks to the hormone progesterone, your intestines are sluggish during pregnancy, which can cause bloating, cramping, and the urge to break wind. Help yourself (and your family!) out by eating gassy foods, such as broccoli, Brussels sprouts, beans, cabbage, cauliflower, corn, and onions, in moderation.

Q. Why am I snoring like a chainsaw?

A. Swollen mucous membranes and congestion can force you to breathe through your mouth and snore, not to mention possibly leaving you with perpetual cold symptoms even though you're not sick. Some strategies: Drink extra fluids; use saline nose drops, especially before you go to sleep; sleep on your left side; run a humidifier; and prop yourself up on some extra pillows.

Q. Why are my nipples as big as dinner plates?

A. Skin darkening caused by hormones may make it look like your nipple is taking over your breast—some say this is nature's way of helping your little one spot his target. Tiny bumps may also sprout around the edges and secrete fluid, helping to keep the stretched-out skin lubricated. Forgo topless sunbathing for the duration, as sun exposure can make the hyperpigmentation permanent. Your areolas will shrink in size when you're finished nursing.

Q. What's up with this drooling?

A. For reasons that are not understood, some pregnant women produce excess saliva—up to three or four quarts a day! Carry a small towel with you in a waterproof tote bag for discreet spitting. Limiting starch in your diet and drinking more water may help. Hard candies can ease the extra swallowing you might be doing, but avoid sour flavors, which can exacerbate the problem.

Q. Why do I leak when I laugh?

A. Laughing (and sneezing) are risky business now that you're drinking about 64 ounces (1.9 l) of fluids a day and you've got an extra 10 pounds (4.5 kg) or so of baby and uterus sitting on your bladder. Make it a point to pee—frequently. The more often you go, the less you'll be holding in when the punch line of the joke hits. Oh, and don't forget to do your Kegels (see page 52).

Q. What is the deal with all this sweat?

A. Perspiration pours from your underarms, between your legs, down your belly, even on your face! Blame the extra blood pumping through and warming your skin. Sweat is your body's way of cooling off. Dress in layers, apply antiperspirant and talc-free powder liberally, and, yes, drink more fluids.

Q. Why do my legs look like a road map?

A. Those enlarged, bulging, purple or black veins in your legs and even labia are varicose veins. To ease the swelling, avoid standing for extended periods, prop your legs up when you can, and avoid crossing them. Also try support hose. When varicose veins occur in your anus, they're called hemorrhoids. A sitz bath can help. (For more relief tips, see page 58.)

yeast down there

We hate to tell you this if you're already prone to yeast infections, but pregnancy hormones encourage them. And if you've never had one before, now might be your (un)lucky chance. Report any signs, like itching or discharge, to your doctor.

tag, you're it

Are you finding bits of skin hanging from your breasts, armpits, or neck? Blame the extra hormones combined with friction. Skin tags are harmless, but if they're uncomfortable, consult a dermatologist.

need a doctor?

If you're not already seeing a gynecologist who delivers babies, seek referrals from family, friends, colleagues, and your primary-care physician for an obstetrician. Once you have compiled a list of candidates, you can call the office for some basic information:

❖ How long has the provider been in practice?

❖ Is she board certified?

❖ How many babies has she delivered?

❖ Who will attend the birth if my practitioner is not available?

❖ At what hospital does she deliver?

❖ What are the office hours?

❖ What kind of emergency care is available after hours?

❖ How quickly can I get an appointment—first one, routine visits, unexpected problems?

let's talk

Once you've narrowed your list to a few obstetrician finalists, consider scheduling interviews. Be sure to note how long it takes to get an appointment and how you are treated by the staff. Questions to ask the doctor in person:

❖ How will we work together before, during, and after the birth?

❖ What is your approach to pain management during labor?

❖ Would we work together on a birth plan?

❖ When should I call you about symptoms? Questions?

❖ How often do you perform inductions? Episiotomies? C-sections?

❖ Do you work with a midwife? If so, how do you coordinate care?

Notes

ask a midwife

Some women choose to receive prenatal care from, and even have their baby delivered by, a midwife. Midwives tend to offer more individualized care than doctors, feeling that pregnancy and childbirth are a natural part of life, as opposed to a medical condition. Ask these questions of a potential midwife:

❖ Are you a Certified Nurse Midwife (CNM)? Midwives should be accredited through the American College of Nurse Midwifery (ACNM.org).

❖ Are you affiliated with a hospital, or do you work out of a freestanding birthing center?

❖ Do you have physician backup in case of an emergency?

the lowdown on checkups

insurance review

Before you go to the first prenatal appointment, it's a good idea to review your health insurance policy to confirm what it covers. Call the company if anything is unclear. Also, talk to your doctor's office about what you will need to pay. Check on items such as:

❖ Your obstetrician

❖ Prenatal visits

❖ Routine tests

❖ The laboratory

❖ Optional tests, such as amniocentesis (see page 108)

❖ Midwife care

❖ Your hospital

❖ Anesthesia during labor and delivery

❖ Delivery and postpartum care (for you)

❖ Postnatal care (for your baby)

❖ Circumcision

Once you confirm your pregnancy, schedule your first prenatal checkup, which usually takes place between weeks 6 and 10. If you're seeing the obstetrician for the first time, you'll fill out a medical history. Be sure to ask the questions on page 102 so you can get to know her philosophies on prenatal care and delivery. You'll also have a pelvic exam, a Pap smear, and blood tests (see page 106). You may even have a transvaginal ultrasound to check your baby's size—and see and hear the heartbeat!

Get used to peeing in a cup—you'll need to do a urine test at each prenatal visit. And, of course, you'll also be weighed and have your blood pressure checked. Expect monthly doctor visits throughout the second trimester; twice a month from weeks 28 to 36, and then weekly until you deliver.

How was your first prenatal visit?

_____

_____

_____

Questions to ask your doctor next time:

_____

_____

_____

_____

_____

Notes

routine tests

FIRST TRIMESTER

urine test

- ❖ **who** all women
- ❖ **when** prenatal visits
- ❖ **how** urine sample

- ❖ **why** To check protein and sugar levels and to detect any urinary tract infections.

anemia

- ❖ **who** all women
- ❖ **when** some prenatal visits
- ❖ **how** blood test

- ❖ **why** To screen for anemia. If you have anemia, your doctor may prescribe iron supplements.

Rh factor

- ❖ **who** all women
- ❖ **when** first prenatal visit
- ❖ **how** blood test

- ❖ **why** To determine your Rh factor, a blood protein. If you're Rh-negative and your baby is Rh-positive, your body will produce antibodies in future pregnancies. Injections administered during pregnancy and after delivery prevent this type of reaction.

rubella immunity

- ❖ **who** all women
- ❖ **when** first prenatal visit
- ❖ **how** blood test

- ❖ **why** To detect antibodies to rubella (German measles), which indicate immunity to the disease. You may not be immune any longer (even if you got the vaccine as a kid), and exposure during the first trimester can cause birth defects.

STDs

- ❖ **who** all women
- ❖ **when** first prenatal visit
- ❖ **how** blood tests and swabs of the vagina and cervix

- ❖ **why** To prevent spreading infection to your baby. Gonorrhea, chlamydia, or syphilis can be treated with antibiotics. Antiviral medication can help control herpes. Medication can decrease the risk of HIV transmission from mother to baby.

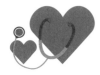

hepatitis B

- ❖ **who** all women
- ❖ **when** usually in the first trimester
- ❖ **how** blood test

- ❖ **why** To check for the hepatitis B virus (HBV), which can put your baby at risk of liver disease. If you're infected, your newborn will be treated and vaccinated soon after birth.

SECOND TRIMESTER

glucose screening

- ❖ **who** all women
- ❖ **when** weeks 24 to 28
- ❖ **how** a blood test done one hour after you drink a sugary liquid

- ❖ **why** To measure blood-sugar level, which indicates the risk of gestational diabetes. If the result is positive, you'll have a follow-up test. Treatment may include diet, exercise, or medication.

THIRD TRIMESTER

group B strep (GBS)

- ❖ **who** all women
- ❖ **when** weeks 35 to 37
- ❖ **how** cells are swabbed from the rectum and vagina

- ❖ **why** To screen for Group B streptococcus (GBS) bacteria, which, if passed to the baby during delivery and not treated, can cause severe illness. If positive, you'll receive antibiotics during delivery.

ANY TIME

ultrasound

- ❖ **who** all women
- ❖ **when** any point in your pregnancy

- ❖ **how** sound waves make a picture of the baby; it can be performed transvaginally or externally
- ❖ **why** To monitor high-risk pregnancies, check the size and position of the fetus and placenta, gauge the amount of amniotic fluid, or look for the presence of multiples.

optional tests

first trimester screen (nuchal translucency)

❖ **who** all women

❖ **when** weeks 11 to 14

❖ **how** blood test combined with an ultrasound that measures the fluid at the back of the baby's neck

❖ **why** To identify risk for Down syndrome, trisomy 18, and heart defects. *Note:* This combined *screening* test has about an 85 percent accuracy rate for identifying these specific chromosomal abnormalities, but it is not a *diagnostic* test (see page 16)! Up to 5 percent of the time, women will test as high-risk when in fact, their pregnancies are normal.

triple/quad (maternal serum) screen

❖ **who** all women

❖ **when** weeks 16 to 18

❖ **how** blood test

❖ **why** To identify risk for Down syndrome and neural tube defects, like spina bifida and anencephaly. The triple screen measures the levels of three pregnancy hormones; the quadruple screen checks four. The two tests are 70 to 80 percent accurate. *Note:* This is a not a *diagnostic* test (see page 16). No more than 5 percent of women who test positive will be carrying a baby with Down syndrome.

chorionic villus sampling (CVS)

❖ **who** women over 35, couples at risk for or with a family history of birth defects, or anyone who receives a positive test result from a first-trimester screen

❖ **when** weeks 10 to 12

❖ **how** a doctor inserts a thin tube into the uterus through the vagina or into the belly to take a sample of placenta tissues

❖ **why** To detect chromosomal disorders, such as Down syndrome, and genetic disorders, such as cystic fibrosis and sickle-cell anemia. *Note:* 1 in 100 procedures may result in a miscarriage.

amniocentesis

❖ **who** women over 35, those with a family history of genetic disorders, or anyone who receives a positive test result from the first-trimester or triple/quad screenings

❖ **when** weeks 15 to 20

❖ **how** a doctor guides a needle through the mother's abdomen and uterus to withdraw amniotic fluid

❖ **why** To diagnose Down syndrome, neural tube defects, and other chromosomal and genetic abnormalities. The test also confirms your baby's gender. Results are 99 percent accurate. *Note:* As many as 1 in 200 to 400 procedures may result in a miscarriage.

Notes

go FISH

Both amniocentesis and CVS test results take between ten days and two weeks. If you'd like to get information faster, there is an add-on test called "FISH" (fluorescent in situ hybridization) that in just a day can diagnose major genetic disorders, including Down syndrome.

not stressing

Performed anytime during the last trimester to monitor the well-being of the fetus, a non-stress test measures fetal heart-rate patterns in women with high-risk pregnancies. A biophysical profile combines a non-stress test with a detailed ultrasound to look at such factors as heart-rate activity, body movements, and the volume of amniotic fluid.

take note *Depending on your age and medical history, many pregnancy tests are optional. Some carry risks, too. Talk with your partner and doctor to decide which ones are right for you.*

pick a pediatrician

The choice of a pediatrician is important—you'll be seeing a lot of each other during your baby's first year and beyond! Once you've lined up some referrals from family, friends, colleagues, and your ob-gyn, you may want to visit and interview a few practitioners before making your final selection. Also take into account factors such as location and insurance coverage. You can start by calling the office to find out basic information, such as:

❖ Length of time the doctor has been practicing and whether she's board certified or has areas of specialization

❖ Office hours, including evenings and weekends

❖ Availability of after-hours advice from a doctor or nurse via telephone or e-mail

❖ Length of time it takes to get a well-baby or last-minute appointment

❖ Average wait times at scheduled appointments

❖ Routine visit and vaccination schedules

❖ Billing and insurance procedures

❖ Availability and cost (if any) of an appointment to interview the doctor in person or by telephone

the little things

When you visit a potential pediatrician's office, take note of the details: the receptionist's demeanor; the cleanliness of the waiting area; hand-sanitizer dispensers; the presence of toys, books, and small furniture for children; and posted info about topics such as immunization, disease prevention, and parenting classes.

If there are other parents in the waiting area (and they seem receptive), ask them what they like or dislike about the practice.

like-minded

When interviewing a pediatrician, ask questions that will give you a sense of her style and whether you will work well together. In case your time with the doctor is limited, ask what's most important to you first, for example: How will I know when to call or bring the baby in? What's your philosophy about breastfeeding and bottle-feeding? What's your recommendation for getting a newborn to sleep?

Notes

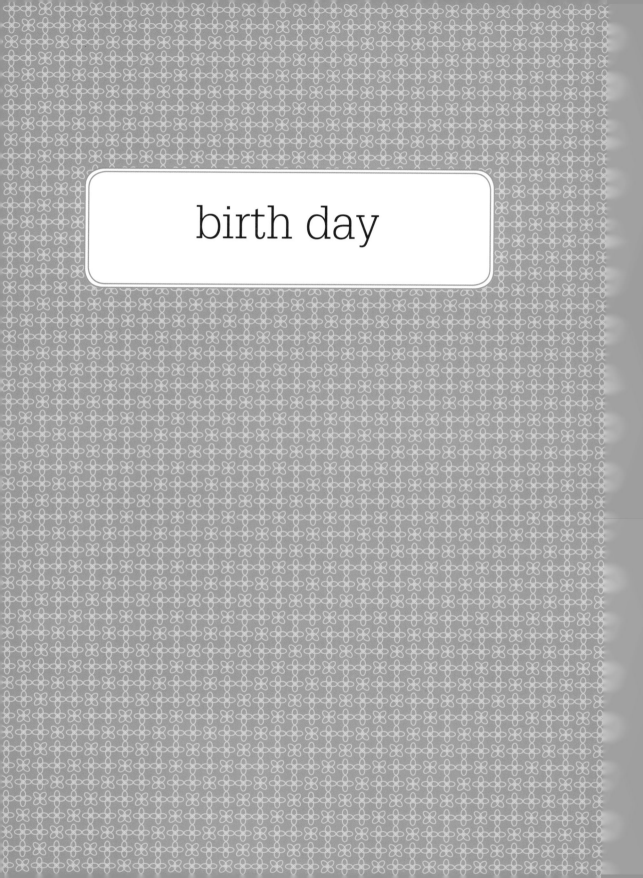

birth day

birth day

Think of it as a trip to a foreign land: Preparing for birth requires advance research, choosing traveling guides and companions, taking a class or two on the subject, making a plan (if that's your style), and packing a bag.

Globe-trotting metaphors aside, whether you feel excited, terrified, or both about childbirth—whether the women in your family are known to labor for days or so quickly that the baby is born in the backseat—it's natural to want to have things go your way. The reality is, though, that many aspects of labor and delivery are out of anyone's control. What you can do is educate yourself about the labor and delivery process and your options, and take steps to help you feel confident that you'll be surrounded by caring health-care professionals. Then remember that whatever happens, at the end of the day (or days), you'll have a baby to show for all your hard work!

What are your hopes about giving birth?

_____

_____

_____

_____

What are your fears about giving birth?

_____

_____

_____

_____

childbirth: the reality

While every woman's labor experience is unique, it always includes three basic stages:

LABOR

Contractions help the cervix to efface (thin out) and dilate (open) to eventually form a birth canal that's 10 centimeters wide. While the cervix is dilating, the contractions are also moving your baby deeper into your pelvis. This first stage of childbirth is generally the longest, with three phases (see chart at right)—each feels very different from the others. (You can use the log on page 123 to time your contractions once they've started.)

DELIVERY

You're completely dilated: Time to push! Contractions of early labor slow to 2 to 5 minutes apart and are accompanied by the uncontrollable urge to bear down. The baby moves through the birth canal until her head begins to crown at the opening of your vagina. This phase could take thirty minutes, or it could last three hours—every woman is different. If it takes a while, you may start to feel discouraged, not to mention exhausted. Hang on! Take encouragement from your birth partner and delivery team, and follow your urge to push.

AFTERBIRTH

Your baby has emerged—but you're not done yet. Your uterus continues to contract to expel the placenta. Then, any tearing or an episiotomy—a small cut made by the doctor to make room for the baby's head—will be stitched up.

why it's called "labor"

	what happens	how you feel	what to do
early phase	Mild contractions occur about 15 to 20 minutes apart and last 30 to 45 seconds, gradually becoming more frequent until they are less than 5 minutes apart and your cervix has dilated to 4 centimeters.	Anywhere from mildly crampy to pretty uncomfortable when a contraction hits.	Call your partner, family, or friends, and put your doctor on alert. Refer to your list of distractions (see page 121), take a shower (or bath, if your water hasn't broken), or go for a walk. Practice your breathing exercises. If you're hungry, eat something light.
active phase	Contractions become more intense and progress from 5 minutes to about 3 minutes apart and 60 seconds long. Your cervix will dilate from 4 to 8 centimeters. Your mucous plug should dislodge and your "bag of waters" (amniotic sac) will break if neither has occurred yet.	Contractions have become more painful now. You may have a hard time breathing through them. You may feel tired between contractions. Many women request pain medication at this point.	Go to the hospital. Change positions and walk around if you're able to, use your breathing techniques to get through contractions, and rest as much as you can in between them. A shower may feel good now.
transition phase	Contractions occur every 2 to 3 minutes and last 60 to 90 seconds as your cervix dilates completely to 10 centimeters.	Contractions are very intense now. You may feel nauseous; have the chills, sweats, or shakes; and begin to feel the urge to push.	Focus on the fact that you're almost there! Switch to rapid pant-blow breathing and try to just ride the waves.

class benefits

Ever wonder how pregnant women managed before the advent of childbirth classes? Sure, it's natural, and, yes, your body will "know what to do." But that doesn't mean it's not enormously helpful to learn about the ins (and outs!) of childbirth beforehand.

The more informed you are, the more relaxed you'll likely be—which could translate into a less painful and scary experience if things don't go as planned. For example, you may not plan to use pain meds, but then change your mind in the thick of things. If you know what to ask for, and the risks and benefits of various options, you're more likely to feel confident about your choices.

class notes

Sometimes all the useful information you hear in classes can be a bit overwhelming, but you know it could come in handy during labor and afterward. Use this space to jot down notes or questions you want to ask at the next session. You can also collect phone numbers and e-mail addresses from your fellow moms-to-be. See page 38 for more on childbirth and parenting classes.

making the call

As you approach your due date, ask your doctor when you should call her. The usual rule of thumb: Make the call when contractions are 5 minutes apart and last about 45 to 60 seconds each, for about an hour. Or pick up the phone when your water breaks if that happens first. (Log your contractions on page 123.)

labor clues

How will you know it's really labor? (It's not like on TV!) As your 40 weeks wind down, be on the alert for:

- ❖ Dropping of the baby's head into the birth canal, or "lightening" (see page 73); it's so-called because you may feel less weighed down once it happens
- ❖ Weight loss of a pound or two
- ❖ Release of the mucous plug
- ❖ Increased pink- or blood-tinged discharge ("bloody show")
- ❖ Diarrhea (the bowels emptying in preparation for delivery)
- ❖ Increased pain in your lower back
- ❖ Menstrual-like cramps
- ❖ Water breaking in a trickle or gush of fluid that is clear and odorless; call your practitioner as soon as this happens
- ❖ True labor contractions (as opposed to Braxton Hicks—see page 62) that are regular, grow closer together, feel stronger, last longer, and don't go away with a change in position

For more details about the stages of labor, see page 114.

it's time to go

You did it all right: You timed your contractions, and you were sure this was it, so you headed to the hospital. Then, after being examined, you're sent home. Don't be embarrassed! It happens often, especially among first-timers.

Research suggests that first-time moms who labor at home until they're in active labor have a lower incidence of interventions, such as c-sections. What's "active" labor? Your contractions will be closer together, and you may find it hard to breathe during a contraction (see page 115). That said, if you live far away from the hospital or your pregnancy has other risk factors, you may want to head out earlier.

what to pack

Don't wait until your due date to pack your hospital bag—babies have a sneaky way of showing up when you least expect them! A few weeks prior, toss some essentials in a small suitcase or duffel. The hospital provides gowns and sanitary pads for you, and diapers, T-shirts, a cap, and swaddling blankets for your baby. You bring the rest. Tip: Attach a list of last-minute items to your bag so you can toss 'em in as you head out the door. Be sure to take:

O Health-insurance card and birth plan (if you wrote one)

O Robe, socks, and slippers

O 2 nursing bras

O Toiletries, such as toothpaste and toothbrush, hair ties and brush, deodorant, and contact lens solution

O Labor aids you may want, including lip balm, lozenges, lollipops, massage lotion, a tennis ball, or an MP3 player with relaxing music

O Video camera and/or digital camera, with memory cards and chargers (or a film camera with lots of film)

O Cell phone (make sure the hospital allows them) and charger

O Going-home clothes for you (yes, that still means maternity clothes!)

O Going-home outfit for your baby

O Post-delivery snacks (you will be starving!) and coins for vending machines

O *Parenting Pregnancy Planner* and a pen

carry-on bag

Your partner's along for the ride, too, so have him pack a bag with a change of clothes, toiletries, and snacks, in case labor lasts a long time. You don't want your significant other in the cafeteria when it's time for the big moment!

what not to pack

❖ Jewelry

❖ Candles (an open flame in a hospital is a no-no)

❖ So much stuff that it clutters up your birthing room and your partner can't carry it all!

119

labor coach

Your go-to labor coach could be your partner, a friend or relative, a midwife, or a doula (see page 54). A team effort works best for some women. Whomever you choose, set aside time before your due date to review notes from your childbirth class together and go over what you want your coach to do. Topics include:

○ The facts about labor, including the stages of labor (page 114) and signs that you are in labor (page 62)

○ How to time contractions (page 123)

○ Instructions on when to go to the hospital (page 118)

○ Breathing techniques you plan to use (practice these together in the weeks leading up to your due date)

○ Your birth preferences or plan; once you're in active labor, you may be too busy or out of breath to voice your wishes yourself

○ Who's allowed in the labor/delivery and postpartum rooms (When it's time to push or, later, to breastfeed, you may not want your entire clan standing around and watching. Your coach can be the one to politely direct traffic.)

sweet somethings

What words or phrases from your labor coach will help you feel confident and reassured during labor? You may already have some favorites that have special meaning to you—or not. Here are a few obvious but useful (you'd be surprised) suggestions.

"You're doing great!"

"Keep breathing."

"Lean on me."

"The baby will be here soon!"

keep the beat

One way or another, your doctor will want to keep tabs on your baby's heart rate during labor and delivery.

❖ Minimally invasive choices include using a handheld ultrasound or stethoscope.

❖ An external fetal monitor wraps around your abdomen and tracks your baby's heart rate and your contractions.

❖ For the clearest readings, especially when your baby's health might be at risk, your doctor may use an internal fetal monitor. Be warned: You'll need to stay in bed.

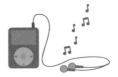

birth-day faves

Jot down what you think will be your favorite pain-relief techniques, labor positions, encouraging phrases, and tips from your childbirth prep classes—the tools you want to remember to use during labor and delivery.

or just scream…

Here are a few go-to tactics for getting through childbirth:

❖ Breathing techniques: Try one, try them all, and try again!

❖ Walk as much as possible.

❖ Try different positions, such as squatting, kneeling, or lying on your side.

❖ Listen to music.

❖ Take a shower.

❖ Have your partner apply firm pressure on your lower back/ sacrum.

❖ Sit, bounce, or just lean on a birthing ball.

❖ Slow dance (giving you a body to lean on and a reason to keep your hips moving).

❖ Meditate or use other relaxation techniques.

your childbirth wish list

Even though "birth" and "plan" don't always go together, many moms-to-be put their ideal game plan on paper. This can be anything from a list of preferences (you do or don't want an epidural) to a detailed point-by-point of how you'd like the birth to go. Discuss your birth preferences with your health-care provider and partner and check with the hospital about what's allowed. Be prepared to change your mind, or have circumstances change it for you. Remember that a healthy mother—yes, you!—and a healthy baby are what's most important.

Some options you might want to consider include:

❖ Who will be present in the delivery room (for example, any family members and friends)

❖ Electronic fetal monitoring (see page 120)

❖ Nonmedical pain relief, such as a shower, a birthing ball, breathing techniques, or massage

❖ Medical pain relief, such as an epidural

❖ Interventions: how you feel about induction, episiotomy, forceps or vacuum extraction, and cesarean section

❖ Religious or spiritual practices

❖ Who will cut the umbilical cord

satisfaction not guaranteed

In a *Babytalk* magazine survey, 70 percent of moms-to-be created a birth plan, but only 16 percent of mothers felt their delivery matched their birth plan.

Eighty-four percent had some surprise, whether she was delivered by a doctor or midwife, and whether her partner was her only coach or she had the help of a doula.

The upshot? Making a birth plan is a good way to go over options and consider possibilities but don't expect things to go exactly as planned when delivery day arrives.

contraction log

	start time	end time	duration	frequency
1				
2				
3				
4				
5				
6				
7				
8				
9				
10				
11				
12				
13				
14				
15				
16				
17				
18				
19				
20				
21				
22				
23				
24				
25				
26				
27				
28				
29				
30				
31				
32				

about time

Timing contractions using a watch or clock with a second hand helps you assess how your labor is progressing and when to head to the hospital.

The number of seconds between the start time and the end time of a contraction is its *duration*. The number of minutes between the start time of one contraction and the start of the next is the *frequency* of contractions.

Usually your doctor will ask you to call when contractions last about 45 to 60 seconds each and are 5 minutes apart, for a period of an hour.

spreading the news

gossip girl

When you're en route to the hospital, you won't have time to call everyone on your speed dial to give them the news. Consider setting up a phone tree, where you can call one or two key people, who in turn have instructions to notify a bunch of others, and so on, and so on. You can also ask your key contacts to send out a group e-mail.

Whichever option you choose, be sure everyone knows the drill—and has current telephone numbers and e-mail addresses.

name	contact info

birth announcement list

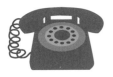

name	sent ✓

here's johnny!

Your friends and family may have gotten that "baby's on the way" call or e-mail, and you can bet that all of them will be eagerly awaiting news of the arrival, as well as time, length and weight stats, and the name of your little one. Oh, and they also want to see a photo, thanks very much.

Have your partner, a relative, or a friend upload a picture, add the relevant info, and send the message to your prepared e-mail list. Later, you can create printed announcements if that's more your style. You may want to address and stamp envelopes now, if you have time on your hands waiting for the big event.

thanks for the memories

write now

The details of your child's birth—when you first realized you were in labor, how contractions felt, what your baby looked like when you first held her in your arms—are precious and fleeting memories.

You may think you'll never forget exactly how it all went down, but the sleep deprivation of the early months of parenthood can leave you racking your brain. Was it 2 P.M. when you dashed to the hospital? How long did you push?

While it's still fresh in your mind, write about it, so you can tell your child the story later on and reminisce with your partner, too.

When did you go into labor? Where were you? What were you doing? Who did you call?

_____

_____

_____

_____

What did contractions feel like? What did you do during and between contractions?

_____

_____

_____

_____

What else happened during labor? When did you go to the hospital? How long were you in labor?

_____

_____

_____

_____

_____

_____

Did anything unusual or unexpected occur?

_____

_____

_____

_____

What happened right after the birth?

_____

_____

_____

_____

_____

What were your first impressions of your baby?

_____

_____

_____

_____

homecoming

homecoming

For some new parents, there's a bizarre moment when you're discharged from the hospital, and you're looking over your shoulder, sure someone's going to stop you from leaving with your baby. What would make them think you're capable of taking care of this teeny, tiny person? Relax: The fact is, a lot of newborn care is instinctual, so try to trust yourself and accept help from anyone who offers—and don't be shy about asking. You and your baby will learn from each other. (Forget housework: Just hang out in bed with your baby and savor your time together.)

Too bad it's not all about getting to know, live with, and care for your pint-size new roommate. The early days of motherhood are complicated by fluctuating hormones, learning to breastfeed, and coping with sleep deprivation. You'll have plenty of "Ick, what's that?" moments as your body recovers from childbirth. So whether you're blissfully cocooning with your baby or feeling somewhat less positive about the whole scene, this chapter will guide you through welcoming home your here-at-last baby.

How does being a mom feel? Is it what you expected?

What are the best parts?

breast issues

Breastfeeding can be deeply satisfying. It can also be frustrating and filled with pitfalls. Here are some ways to cope:

❖ **Engorgement**. If your breasts are painful, hard, and tight when your milk comes in, nurse frequently and use cold compresses between feedings. Pumping briefly may provide some relief, but too much pumping can also exacerbate the problem.

❖ **Painful nipples**. Your nipples may be sensitive for days or even weeks. Cracked and sore nipples are common. Apply pure-lanolin ointment often. Call your doctor if symptoms worsen.

❖ **Forceful letdown**. If your milk sprays or shoots out too quickly, try gently expressing milk manually or briefly pump some milk before offering the breast.

❖ **Thrush**. You can get a yeast infection on your nipples or even in your breasts, where you may feel sharp pain during or after nursing. Symptoms include extremely sore or burning nipples, which may also be red or itchy. Contact your doctor right away; treatments include a topical or oral medication.

❖ **Blocked duct**. A blockage may feel like a knot under the skin. To help prevent blocked ducts, alternate your baby's position at each feeding. If you have a blocked duct, gently massage the area and apply warm compresses before and while nursing. After nursing, cold compresses may offer relief. Nurse often, and use a pump, if needed, to help empty the affected breast.

❖ **Mastitis**. If you suddenly have a high fever, plus body aches, chills, headache, or more fatigue than usual, you might have a breast infection, which can appear with almost no warning. Call your doctor, who may prescribe antibiotics. Meanwhile, you can take acetaminophen or ibuprofen for the pain and fever. Also try to nurse often, even if your milk supply is decreased.

❖ **Raynaud's syndrome**. If you have severe, throbbing pain in your nipples, it could be Raynaud's syndrome, which is often misdiagnosed as a yeast infection. If you have this condition, small arteries in the nipples constrict and the skin blanches when you nurse. Talk to your doctor for treatment.

latch on

When your baby's mouth isn't locked on properly, soreness can result—as well as a hungry baby! Her mouth should cover as much of the areola as possible—not just your nipple. If she misses, break the seal by gently slipping your pinky into the corner of her mouth and try again. See just how it's done by watching the latching-on video at Parenting.com.

cabbage patch

To reduce pain from engorgement or mastitis, try putting refrigerated green cabbage leaves on your breast. Apply for no more than 20 minutes, twice a day. Any more than that could cause your milk supply to decrease.

taking care of you

Your baby takes priority, of course, but don't forget to care for yourself, too! These tips will keep your energy and your spirits up:

❖ Shower and dress when you can. You may not feel up to it, and you may not get to do it until dinnertime, but you'll feel better.

❖ Try to get outside for some fresh air and, if possible, a walk.

❖ Don't expect to fit into pre-baby clothes anytime soon (see page 136), so focus on dressing in comfy clothes that make it easier to nurse and to grab a nap when the opportunity arises.

❖ Screen your calls; limit visitors to those who will lend a hand.

❖ Connect with moms who have babies the same age as yours. Ask each other questions, laugh, cry. You'll find plenty online, and some mothers' groups form naturally, for instance, out of a birth class. Organizations, such as hospitals and parents' clubs, also sponsor them. Some moms stay close to their mothers' group pals for life.

poop notes

Along with monitoring your baby's weight, tracking the frequency of feedings and diaper changes will help you and your pediatrician know whether your newborn is getting enough to eat.

Lucky you: The color and consistency of baby poop is also important. The doctor will ask for this information during the early visits. *Tip:* Check out "The Ultimate Guide to Poop" at Parenting.com.

newborn body care

Your newborn can have only sponge baths for the first week or two, until her umbilical cord stump falls off. Even after that, you don't actually have to bathe her very often. Wiping her bottom clean during diaper changes and sponge bathing her two or three times a week is plenty. (See page 83 for tub supplies.)

Keep the umbilical cord area dry. Fold down the top of the diaper and keep clothes loose over this area. There's no need to swab it with rubbing alcohol. In a week or two, it'll fall off on its own.

When her nails get long or if, like many babies, yours comes out of the womb with long fingernails, trim them with baby-size nail clippers or scissors. (This may be easiest while she is sleeping.) Otherwise she could scratch herself.

| take note | *If breastfeeding does not go smoothly for you, get help right away. Don't wait! Talk to your doctor, a lactation consultant, and veteran moms. Also check out local breastfeeding support groups.* |

growth chart

date	weight	length

well-baby visits

The first trip to the pediatrician will likely take place within a few days of bringing your baby home. You'll be back again in two weeks, and then at one- or two-month intervals for the first six months. At each appointment, the doctor or a nurse will listen to his heartbeat; perform a physical exam; check and plot on a graph your baby's weight and length; talk to you about his eating and sleeping habits; and answer your questions.

According to the schedule recommended by the American Academy of Pediatrics, vaccinations start with a Hepatitis B vaccine before your newborn leaves the hospital, with a second dose one to two months later, and a final one after 24 weeks. Other vaccines will then follow at specific intervals.

Notes

_____

_____

_____

_____

_____

_____

_____

_____

_____

_____

_____

_____

sleep, baby, sleep

The irony: Your new family member finally arrives, and all you want is for her to sleep. While newborns typically will snooze 16 hours or more each day, it's broken up in fits and spurts by frequent feedings and diaper changes.

Try to put her down about every two hours after feeding and burping—immediately if she acts sleepy. Rubbing her eyes, yawning, or fussing are all cues that she's past due for a nap. It's fine to use whatever works to get a newborn to nod off. Tried-and-true approaches include walking, swaddling, and singing. It's okay if she falls asleep in a bouncy seat or a swing—just don't leave her unattended.

mom to mom

"I love the little looks she gives me when she is about to nurse. She gives me this indescribable look that only I get to see. She gets so excited and starts kicking and throwing her arms everywhere with a giant smile on her face."

"ick! what's that?" the postpartum version

The postpartum recovery period (about six weeks after vaginal birth, or up to eight weeks after a c-section) is full of dramatic, and sometimes weird, physical and emotional changes. Every mom's experience is different, but here's a hint of what to expect:

❖ **Afterpains**. These period-like cramps occur as the uterus shrinks back down to its original size. For relief, try gently massaging your belly, applying heat, emptying your bladder often, and taking acetaminophen or ibuprofen.

❖ **Baby blues**. It's estimated that more than half of women feel an emotional letdown after birth. The shift in hormones added to round-the-clock demands of childcare can cause moodiness, irritability, and sadness lasting for weeks. To cope, try to get outside with your baby each day, seek support from other moms (see page 131), and hand the baby over to someone else when you need (or want) a break.

❖ **Breast tenderness/engorgement**. If you're breastfeeding, your boobs are on a wild ride for the first week or two. Your milk may take a few days to come in, and then you may end up engorged, and your nipples are likely to be sore. (For helpful tips, see page 130.)

❖ **Constipation**. Your bowels will be sluggish. Try drinking more fluids, eating a fiber-rich diet, and getting some gentle exercise. Check with your doctor about taking a stool softener.

❖ **Depression**. For about 10 to 20 percent of new mothers, the so-called "baby blues" may develop into postpartum depression. Symptoms include persistent feelings of guilt, inadequacy, or extreme sadness; difficulty concentrating; sleeping or eating problems; and apathy toward the baby. If you think you might be depressed, seek help immediately—it is not a sign of failure! Your doctor can prescribe medication (some can be taken safely while nursing) or refer you to a mental-health professional.

❖ **Hair loss**. Finding clumps of hair in the drain? It's normal to shed the hair you held on to during pregnancy. It'll stabilize as your hormones settle down.

- **Hemorrhoids**. These inflamed rectal veins can result from the strain of pushing during delivery. They typically improve in a few weeks. Soothe them with cold witch hazel compresses or warm baths. Kegel exercises will speed healing (see page 52).

- **Increased perspiration**. Night sweats can last a few weeks as your body sheds excess fluid (and weight!). Sleep on a towel, wear cotton pj's, and keep a spare pair of pj's near the bed.

- **Lochia**. This is essentially a period that lasts weeks as your uterus sheds its lining. The discharge will be heavy and bright red for a few days and then lighten and turn brownish. Use sanitary pads (not tampons). Call your doctor if the discharge turns red and gets heavier again (you could be overdoing it!).

- **Loose abdomen**. The ab muscles that stretched to make room for the baby may remain loose, leaving you more vulnerable to back strain. They will shrink (almost) back to normal, but be gentle with them now, especially when lifting.

- **Perineal pain**. The skin and muscles between your vagina and rectum may be tender from an episiotomy, tearing, or stretching. Reduce the initial swelling with ice packs. Sitz baths, warm compresses, and acetaminophen or ibuprofen can also help. To prevent infection, rinse and dry after using the toilet; you can use a hair dryer set on low. Sit on soft surfaces, such as a donut pillow, and try doing Kegel exercises.

- **Sleep deprivation**. Don't underestimate how hard lack of sleep can be on your emotional state and your relationship with your partner. The best advice: "Sleep when the baby sleeps." (Even though it's hard when there's so much laundry to do!)

- **Urinary problems**. If peeing is difficult, try running water to help inspire a flow to get started. If incontinence is your issue, empty your bladder often and do some Kegels. Call your doctor if symptoms don't improve within a few weeks.

mommy tummy

Your doctor can tell you if your outer ab muscles split during pregnancy (*diastasis recti*), and, if so, what you can do to speed healing: physical therapy, a tummy splint, or gentle exercises. Don't do sit-ups or crunches! They can widen the split, as can motions—twisting, lifting, bending—that put pressure on your outer abs. Focus on toning your transverse abdominal muscle, instead.

Once your doctor gives the okay, try gentle pelvic tilts to strengthen your transverse ab muscle. Lie on your back with knees bent and feet on the floor. Breathe in deeply, expanding your abdomen. As you exhale, bring your belly button back to your spine and hold, pressing your back to the floor. Aim for a set of ten tilts daily. (Also see page 58.)

the new normal

Whether you lose all your pregnancy weight in six weeks or six months or a year, it's unlikely your body will ever be exactly the same (no matter what the celeb magazines show!). Expect a new kind of normal, which may include increases—or decreases—in your waistline, hips, butt, and bust measurements, as well as some scars, stretch marks, and belly button stretching.

It took nine months to put all that weight on, so expect and allow at least nine months to take it off. Now isn't the time to scrimp on nutrients! Every new mom needs to keep her energy humming, and if you're nursing, you need an extra 500 calories a day.

ease into exercise

Your body has been through a lot. No matter what number is on the scale or how soft your belly looks, resist the temptation to jump into a rigorous exercise routine. With the approval of your doctor, start with short walks, gentle stretching, and pelvic tilts (see page 135) to improve abdominal tone.

At about six weeks, if your ob-gyn says it's safe and you feel up to it, you may want to step up your routine. Take longer walks, or try out a postnatal aerobics, yoga, or pilates class, DVD, or podcast. Mom-and-baby exercise classes or a stroller-walking group will help you tone up and meet other moms in the same boat.

Exercise can also be welcome alone time. Schedule your workout for just after you nurse. Head to the gym or pool, go to a class, or just jog around the neighborhood at your own pace.

who has time for sex?

While your ob-gyn may clear you physically for having sex at your six-week postpartum checkup, that won't necessarily mean you'll feel like doing it. Hormone levels drop at delivery, quashing your libido, and breastfeeding hormones may leave you, uh, a bit dry. Add sore, leaky breasts, a still-tender perineum, and exhaustion, and you may not yet be ready to get it on.

take it slow

When you do decide you're ready, go easy on yourself. Ask your partner to be extra gentle and use lots of lubricant. And don't forget birth control—unless you want to have another baby right away. Breastfeeding is not a foolproof form of birth control. Even if your period has not returned, you can still ovulate.

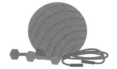

postpartum visit

Your postpartum checkup will typically take place six weeks after birth. If you've had a c-section, you'll be seen earlier so that your ob-gyn can check your incision. During the appointment, she will examine your uterus and vagina, inspecting any stitches and tears for proper healing. Your doctor will also check your breasts for signs of infection. This is a good time to discuss any concerns you have about sex, birth control, weight loss, exercise, your emotions, and persistent symptoms, such as fatigue.

Notes

index

notes and to-dos

key contacts

Physician _____

_____

Insurance _____

_____

Pharmacy _____

_____

Hospital _____

_____

Pediatrician _____

_____

Other _____

_____

_____

_____

_____

_____

Claim your subscription to *Parenting Early Years* now!

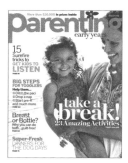

Thank you for your purchase of *Parenting's Pregnancy Planner*. Included is a one-year subscription (11 issues valued at $10) to *Parenting Early Years* magazine.

Parenting Early Years is specifically tailored for moms of children age 0 to 5.

Fill out and mail this paid subscription voucher to begin receiving your subscription to *Parenting Early Years*.

How this Promotion Works:

Included with your purchase of *Pregnancy Planner* for $19.95 is a one-year (11 issue, $10.00 value) subscription to *Parenting Early Years* magazine. Fill in your name and address and mail to:

> Parenting Magazine Liaison
> Attn: Parenting Pregnancy Planner
> Palm Coast Data
> PO Box 420235
> Palm Coast, FL 32142-0235

Yes! Start my subscription to *Parenting Early Years*.

Name _____

Address _____

City / State / Zip _____

XJ0PPB

Terms & Conditions:

If you're already a *Parenting*® subscriber, a one-year extension to your subscription will be included with your $19.95 purchase of *Pregnancy Planner*. There are no hidden charges or automatic renewals. You will never receive a bill for this subscription. Please allow 6–8 weeks for delivery of your first issue.

Offer valid for US subscribers only. Limit one subscription per household, family, or address. Offer expires December 31, 2011. Please note that your name and address that you provide will be handled in accordance with *Parenting's* privacy policy which can be found at http://www.parenting.com/article/Parenting/Customer-Service/Privacy-Policy. If you prefer not to receive this magazine and would like a rebate for the value instead, please PRINT the word "rebate" on this form, fill in the information above, and mail it along with a copy of your purchase receipt within 30 days of purchasing the book. Your rebate will not be processed without valid proof of purchase. Checks will be sent within 12 weeks of receipt of request.

Other Restrictions:

Limit one promotional subscription per customer per household/family per address. We reserve the right to end the promotion at any time.

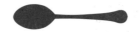
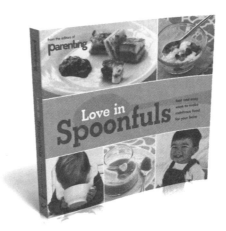